Copyright Page
Less Sugar, More Focus
© 2025 Ivelisse Adorno

First edition published in 2025
Published by Kitvi Editorial, LLC
www.iveadorno.com

The content of this book is for informational purposes only and is based on the author's personal experience, knowledge, and research. It is not intended to replace professional medical advice. Please consult with a healthcare professional before making significant changes to your diet.

For permissions, collaborations, or institutional distribution:
libros@iveadorno.com

Table of Content

Introduction

Eating and nourishing are not the same.

Eating can be a response to hunger, routine, or cravings; nourishing, on the other hand, is a conscious act of love and responsibility toward our body. As temples of the Spirit, caring for what we consume carries not only physical but also spiritual implications. Eating well is a way to honor the life we've been given and to align ourselves with God's divine purpose of health and wholeness.

This book was born out of a deeply personal journey. For years, I struggled with brain fog, exhaustion, anxiety, and a sense of disconnection from my own body. It was a process marked by trial and error, tears, learning, and faith. What you'll find in these pages is not a distant theory or passing trend–it's the fruit of a real transformation, shared with honesty, compassion, and hope.

In recent years, science has confirmed what many of us already sensed: excess sugar doesn't only affect the body–it clouds the mind. Studies have shown that diets high in added sugars can negatively impact memory, concentration, and decision-making. Research published in *Neuroscience* and *Nutritional Neuroscience* has linked excessive glucose intake to brain inflammation, cognitive decline, and reduced emotional regulation. It's also been found that high-sugar diets can alter gut microbiota, which directly impacts mood and mental clarity through what is known as the "gut-brain axis."

Blood sugar spikes and crashes affect our daily focus, creating what we call brain fog: that sense of mental sluggishness, low energy, and disorganization. Additionally, studies from UCLA and Harvard have shown that sugar can influence the brain's decision-making centers, making it harder to resist impulses and plan ahead.

That's why this book is not just a recipe guide–it's a tool for renewal. Eating mindfully and reducing sugar intake doesn't only transform your body; it restores the focus, energy, and balance you long for.

For many women, perimenopause, menopause, or diabetes risk present unique physical and emotional challenges. Many men also face metabolic shifts, insulin resistance, or simply wish to optimize their health. This plan is for anyone who wants to live with greater clarity, energy, and purpose.

Less Sugar, More Focus: 30 Days of Low-Carb Meals is more than a cookbook. It's an invitation to rediscover what it means to nourish yourself with intention and to love your body through every decision you make. This approach emphasizes vegetables, clean proteins, healthy fats, and carbs in their most natural forms–supporting a sharper mind and a stronger body.

A low-carb lifestyle can help you:

- Stabilize blood sugar levels
- Reduce systemic inflammation
- Support hormonal health
- Improve digestion and gut microbiota
- Maintain a healthy weight

- Regain energy and mental clarity

As you begin this 30-day journey, you'll see that healthy eating doesn't mean giving up flavor–it means rediscovering it in its most vibrant and healing form. Every recipe is a chance to heal, to focus, and to live with intention.

And the best part? You don't have to do it alone.

Join our private Facebook community, where we walk this journey together:

www.facebook.com/groups/menosazucarmasenfoque

We'll support you with ideas, encouragement, motivation, and unwavering faith that change is possible.

Let's eat less sugar and live with more focus–together!

BREAKFASTS THAT AWAKEN YOUR FOCUS

Start your day by feeding your purpose

BREAKFASTS

Less sugar in the morning. More focus for the rest of the day.

What you choose for breakfast doesn't just affect your stomach–it affects your mind. Starting your day with a low-carb breakfast is a powerful strategy for gaining clarity, sustained energy, and conscious decision-making from the moment you wake up.

When we begin the morning with refined carbohydrates–like white bread, sugary cereals, or baked goods–we trigger a rapid spike in blood sugar levels. That spike is quickly followed by a crash, which leads to fatigue, irritability, early hunger, and brain fog. These glucose highs and lows don't just drain your body–they rob you of focus and productivity.

In contrast, a low-carb breakfast rich in protein, healthy fats, and vegetables stabilizes blood sugar and enhances your ability to concentrate, remember, and exercise self-control. Studies in nutritional neuroscience have shown that elevated sugar levels can negatively impact cognitive function and mood, while a low-sugar diet promotes clearer thinking and sharper focus.

This kind of breakfast is especially powerful for those navigating stages like perimenopause, menopause, diabetes, or insulin resistance. It supports a balanced metabolism and helps avoid the emotional ups and downs that often accompany these conditions.

Moreover, having a sugar-free, intentional breakfast connects you with your purpose from the very first bite. You're not just feeding your body–you're nourishing your focus, your energy, and your daily purpose.

From a spinach and avocado omelet to a green smoothie with plant-based protein, this book offers simple, delicious, and restorative options to help you start the day on the right foot– with a clear mind.

Eat with purpose. Live with focus.

Scrambled Eggs with Spinach and Cheese

Ingredients *(serves 2):*

- 2 large eggs
- 1 cup fresh spinach
- ¼ cup (30 g) shredded cheese (cheddar, mozzarella, or your favorite)
- 1 tablespoon ghee butter or avocado oil
- Salt and pepper to taste – you may also use cumin or dried sofrito for added flavor

Instructions:

1. In a skillet, melt the ghee or heat the avocado oil over medium heat.
2. Add the spinach and cook until tender (about 1-2 minutes).
3. In a bowl, whisk the eggs with a pinch of salt and pepper.
4. Pour the eggs into the skillet with the spinach and stir gently until cooked to your desired consistency.
5. Add the shredded cheese, stir to melt, and serve immediately.
6. Optional: Season with dried sofrito for an extra boost of flavor.

Ham and Mushroom Omelet

Ingredients *(serves 2)*:

- 6 large eggs
- 1 tablespoon Greek yogurt
- 4 oz (about 50 g) of your favorite ham, diced
- 1 cup fresh mushrooms, sliced
- 2 tablespoons butter or avocado oil
- 1 cup (about 30 g) shredded provolone cheese *(optional)*
- Salt and pepper to taste
- Everything Bagel seasoning *(optional)*

Instructions:

1. Heat the butter in a skillet over medium heat.
2. Sauté the mushrooms until golden brown.
3. Add the diced ham and cook for about 1 minute. Remove from the skillet and set aside.
4. In a bowl, whisk the eggs and Greek yogurt with a pinch of salt and pepper.
5. Add a little more butter to the skillet and pour in the egg mixture. Cook over medium-low heat. You may cover the skillet to speed up cooking.

6. Once the eggs are almost fully set, flip the omelet and
    add the ham and mushroom mixture (and the cheese, if
    using).
7. Fold the omelet in half, sprinkle a little cheese on top,
    and cook for one more minute. Serve hot.
8. Garnish with fresh cilantro and Everything Bagel
    seasoning, if desired.

Plain Greek Yogurt with Walnuts and Blueberries

Ingredients *(serves 2):*

- 1½ cups plain unsweetened Greek yogurt, preferably organic
- 1 tablespoon chopped walnuts
- 1 tablespoon fresh blueberries
- 1 teaspoon cranberry seeds
- *Optional:* a few drops of orange extract or sugar-free sweetener

Instructions:

1. Place the Greek yogurt in your favorite bowl.
2. In a skillet over medium heat, toast the walnuts, stirring constantly for 2-3 minutes to bring out their flavor.
3. Sprinkle the chopped walnuts and fresh blueberries over the yogurt.
4. If you prefer a sweeter taste, add a few drops of orange extract or a bit of sugar-free sweetener.
5. Lightly mix and garnish with cranberry seeds.
6. Enjoy this simple and nourishing breakfast!

Baked Egg-Stuffed Avocado

Ingredients *(serves 2)*:

- 2 large avocados, halved and pitted
- 4 small eggs
- Salt, pepper, and your favorite seasonings to taste
- Toasted walnuts
- ½ cup flavored Greek yogurt of your choice
- ¼ cup fresh strawberries

Instructions:

1. Preheat the oven to 350°F (180°C).
2. Scoop out a bit of the avocado flesh to create enough space for the eggs.
3. Place the avocado halves on a baking sheet lined with parchment paper.
4. Crack an egg into a small cup, then gently pour it into the hollow of each avocado half. Season with salt, pepper, and your favorite spices.
5. Bake for 12-15 minutes or until the eggs are cooked to your preferred doneness.
6. Serve warm.

Pair with toasted walnuts, Greek yogurt, and fresh strawberries

Chaffles (Cheese and Egg Waffles)

Ingredients for 2 chaffles:

- 2 large eggs
- 1 cup shredded mozzarella cheese *(you can also use cheddar or a cheese blend, according to your preference)*
- 2 tablespoons almond flour *(optional, for a firmer texture)*
- ½ teaspoon baking powder *(optional, for a fluffier result)*

Instructions:

1. Preheat your waffle maker. Lightly grease it with butter, cooking spray, or oil to prevent sticking. I like to use a bit of bacon grease for added flavor.
2. In a bowl, beat the eggs. Add the shredded cheese, almond flour, and baking powder (if using). Mix well until the ingredients are fully combined into a smooth batter.
3. Pour the batter into the hot waffle maker, making sure not to overfill to avoid overflow. Cook for 3-4 minutes or until golden and crispy.
4. Carefully remove the chaffles and serve them hot. Enjoy them on their own or with your favorite toppings: avocado, salsa, sour cream, or even a touch of honey for a sweet version.

Notes:

- For a sweet twist, add ¼ teaspoon of date sugar, a pinch of cinnamon, and a few drops of vanilla extract to the batter.
- For extra crispiness, let the chaffles cool slightly before serving.

Chia Pudding with Almond Milk and Cinnamon

Ingredients *(serves 2):*

- 3/8 cup chia seeds
- 2 cups unsweetened almond milk
- ½ teaspoon ground cinnamon, or to taste
- *Optional:* 2 dates, for natural sweetness, flavor, and fiber

Instructions:

1. Combine all the ingredients in two containers with lids.
2. Refrigerate for at least 4 hours or overnight, stirring occasionally.
3. Serve cold, and if desired, sprinkle a bit of extra cinnamon on top.
4. You can garnish with fresh strawberries and almonds.
5. At home, we like to add cranberry seeds for a little extra texture and flavor.

Bacon with Fried Eggs and Avocado

Ingredients *(serves 2)*:

- 4 strips of bacon, preferably without added sugars
- 4 large eggs
- Salt and pepper to taste
- 1 ripe avocado
- Macadamia nuts
- 1 chaffle *(optional, for extra protein – see recipe above)*

Instructions:

1. Cook the bacon in a skillet over medium heat until golden and crispy. Remove and set aside.
2. In the same skillet, fry the eggs to your preferred doneness.
3. Serve the fried eggs with hot bacon, half an avocado, and a handful of macadamia nuts.
4. If you're using chaffles, you can make a sandwich and toast it in the skillet with a little butter.

Kale or Romaine Wraps with Ham and Cream Cheese

Ingredients *(serves 2):*

- 4 large leaves of kale or romaine lettuce
- 4 slices of ham (your preferred type)
- 4 tablespoons cream cheese, at room temperature
- 2 dates
- ¼ cup toasted almonds

Instructions:

1. Spread the cream cheese over the lettuce or kale leaves.
2. Place the slices of ham on top and roll them up like a wrap.
3. Serve immediately with a date and toasted almonds on the side.
4. *Optional:* Add scrambled eggs for extra protein.

Cauliflower Toast with Guacamole and Fried Egg

Ingredients *(serves 2):*

- 2 slices of cauliflower "bread"
- 1 serving of guacamole
- 2 fried eggs, cooked to your preference
- Dried sofrito *(optional)*

Instructions:

1. Slice the cauliflower into toast-sized pieces.
2. In a skillet with a bit of butter, toast the cauliflower slices until golden and slightly crispy.
3. Spread guacamole over the cauliflower toast.
4. Top with a fried egg and serve hot.
5. Season with salt, pepper, and dried sofrito, if desired.

Optional add-ons for extra flavor and texture:

- Chopped walnuts or pumpkin seeds for crunch
- A sprinkle of shredded cheese (parmesan, goat cheese, or feta)
- Sliced cherry tomatoes or thinly sliced red onion

Noatmeal (Oatmeal Substitute)

Ingredients *(serves 2):*

- 4 tablespoons chia seeds
- 4 tablespoons almond flour
- 2 tablespoons coconut flour
- 2 tablespoons ground flaxseeds
- 2 cups unsweetened almond milk
- Sweetener to taste *(I use date sugar)*
- Vanilla extract and cinnamon to taste

Instructions:

1. In a saucepan, combine all the ingredients.
2. Cook over medium heat, stirring until the mixture reaches your desired oatmeal-like consistency.
3. Serve warm. You can top it with fresh or dried fruits, nuts, and a sprinkle of cinnamon.

Low-Carb French Toast

Ingredients *(serves 2):*

- 4 slices of low-carb cinnamon bread
- 2 large eggs
- ¼ cup unsweetened almond milk or coconut milk
- ½ teaspoon vanilla extract
- ½ teaspoon ground cinnamon
- ¼ teaspoon sweetener of your choice *(Erythritol, Stevia, Monk Fruit, etc. – I use date sugar)*
- 1 tablespoon butter or coconut oil for cooking

Instructions:

1. In a shallow bowl, whisk together the eggs, almond milk, vanilla, cinnamon, and sweetener.
2. Dip each slice of bread into the mixture, making sure it absorbs well on both sides.
3. Heat a non-stick skillet over medium heat and melt a bit of butter or coconut oil.
4. Place the soaked bread slices in the skillet and cook for 2-3 minutes per side, until golden brown and fully cooked.

To serve:

- Serve the French toast hot, topped with fresh berries, sugar-free syrup or honey, and a sprinkle of cinnamon to taste.

Ham and Cheese Rolls with Avocado

Ingredients *(serves 2):*

- 6 slices of low-carb ham
- 6 slices of your favorite cheese
- 1 avocado, thinly sliced
- Pecans
- Fresh strawberries and blueberries

Instructions:

1. Place a slice of avocado on each piece of ham and cheese.
2. Roll them up and secure with a toothpick if needed.
3. Serve with pecans and fresh fruit on the side.
4. Serve cold.

Spinach and Cheese Frittata

Ingredients *(serves 4):*

- 8 large eggs
- ¼ cup heavy cream or plain Greek yogurt
- 1 cup fresh spinach
- ½ cup sliced mushrooms *(optional)*
- 6 cherry tomatoes, halved
- ¼ cup chopped onion
- ½ cup shredded mozzarella cheese or your preferred cheese
- 2 tablespoons grated Parmesan cheese
- 2 tablespoons olive oil or butter
- Salt, pepper, and paprika to taste

Instructions:

1. Preheat your oven to 375°F (190°C).
2. Wash and chop the spinach, mushrooms, and onion. Grate the cheeses.
3. In an oven-safe skillet, heat the olive oil or butter over medium heat. Add the chopped onion and cook until golden. Then add the mushrooms and cook for about 3 more minutes, until tender. Finally, add the spinach and cherry tomatoes and cook until just wilted.
4. In a large bowl, whisk the eggs with the heavy cream or Greek yogurt. Season with salt and pepper to taste.
5. Pour the egg mixture over the vegetables in the skillet. Make sure everything is evenly distributed. Sprinkle the mozzarella and Parmesan cheese on top.
6. Transfer the skillet to the preheated oven and bake for 12-15 minutes, or until the eggs are fully set and the top is lightly golden.
7. Carefully remove from the oven and let cool slightly. Slice and serve. You can enjoy it with a green salad or fresh avocado.

Egg and Avocado Bowl with Dried Fruit and Nuts

Ingredients *(serves 2):*

- 4 hard-boiled eggs
- 1 avocado, sliced
- Salt and pepper to taste
- Ground cumin (optional, if you like)
- ¼ cup dried fruit

Instructions:

1. In a saucepan, bring water with a splash of vinegar to a boil. Once boiling, reduce to medium heat and gently add the eggs. Cook for about 8 minutes.
2. Transfer the eggs to an ice water bath to cool quickly and make peeling easier.
3. Cut the eggs in half and arrange them in a bowl.
4. Add the avocado slices and season to taste.
5. Finish with a handful of dried fruit and nuts or almonds.

Cream Cheese Pancakes with Caramelized Bacon and Almond Butter Drizzle

Ingredients *(serves 2):*

- 3 eggs
- 6 strips of bacon
- 2 oz cream cheese
- 1 tablespoon almond flour
- 1 teaspoon baking powder
- Cinnamon to taste
- Agave syrup to taste
- ½ teaspoon vanilla extract
- 1 tablespoon unsweetened almond butter

Instructions:

1. Slice the bacon into strips and cook until crispy and golden. Add agave syrup to taste to caramelize. Set aside.
2. In a blender, combine the eggs, cream cheese, almond flour, baking powder, cinnamon, vanilla, and agave. Blend until smooth.
3. In a non-stick skillet over medium-low heat, melt a little butter. Pour the batter into small portions and cook for about 3 minutes on each side until golden. Set aside.
4. Microwave the almond butter for about 15 seconds until melted and pourable.
5. On a plate, stack the pancakes, drizzle with melted almond butter, and top with the caramelized bacon and nuts.
6. Optionally, sprinkle with cinnamon and garnish with a mint leaf or fresh fruit.

Coconut Pancakes with Sugar-Free Syrup

Ingredients *(makes 4 small pancakes):*

- 2 large eggs
- 2 tablespoons coconut flour
- 1 teaspoon baking powder
- 1 tablespoon melted butter
- Sugar-free syrup for serving
- Fresh fruit

Instructions:

1. In a bowl, mix the eggs, coconut flour, baking powder, and melted butter until smooth and well combined.
2. In a non-stick skillet over medium-low heat, melt a little butter. Pour the batter in small portions and cook for about 3 minutes per side, or until golden. Set aside.
3. Serve with sugar-free syrup.
4. Add fresh fruit and nuts if desired.

Poached Eggs with Asparagus

Ingredients *(serves 2):*

- 4 large eggs
- 12 fresh asparagus spears
- 1 tablespoon white vinegar
- Salt and pepper to taste
- Hollandaise sauce *(recipe included below)*

Instructions:

1. Steam the asparagus or cook them in olive oil for extra flavor.
2. Bring water to a gentle boil in a saucepan and add the vinegar.
3. Crack the eggs into the hot water and poach for 3-4 minutes.
4. Serve the poached eggs over the asparagus and season to taste.

Hollandaise Sauce

Ingredients:

- 3 egg yolks
- ½ cup butter (melted and warm)
- 1 tablespoon lemon juice
- Salt and pepper to taste

Instructions:

1. Warm the yolks gently: In a heatproof bowl, add the egg yolks and whisk vigorously.
2. Use a double boiler method: Place the bowl over a pot with hot water (without touching the water). Keep whisking as the yolks warm up, making sure they don't cook or scramble.
3. Add the butter: Slowly pour in the warm melted butter while continuously whisking. The mixture will begin to thicken.
4. Incorporate the lemon juice and season with salt and pepper to taste.

Adjust texture: If the sauce is too thick, add a few drops of hot water while continuing to whisk until smooth.

Cottage Cheese with Strawberries

Ingredients *(serves 2):*

- 1 cup cottage cheese
- 3 strawberries, sliced
- Pistachios

Instructions:

1. Divide the cottage cheese into two bowls.
2. Top with sliced strawberries and pistachios. Serve immediately.

Note: You can add lemon zest to enhance the flavor, and a drizzle of organic honey if desired.

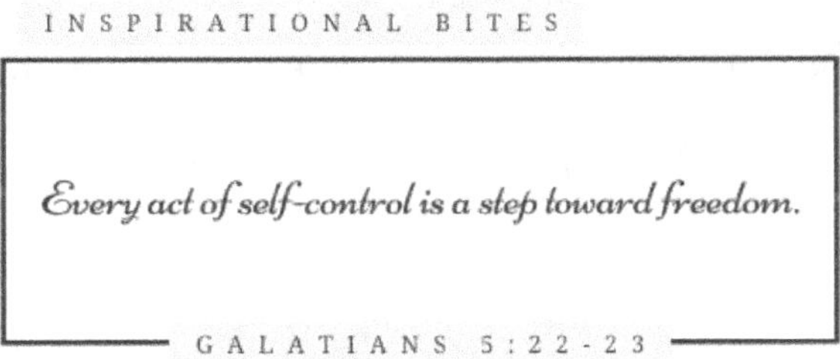

Kale and Feta Scramble

Ingredients *(serves 2):*

- 4 large eggs
- 2 cups chopped kale
- ½ cup crumbled feta cheese
- 1 tablespoon avocado oil
- Salt and pepper to taste
- Paprika for garnish

Instructions:

1. Heat the oil in a skillet over medium heat.
2. Sauté the kale until tender.
3. In a bowl, whisk the eggs with salt and pepper, then pour into the skillet.
4. Cook until the eggs are set, then stir in the feta cheese.
5. Sprinkle with paprika and serve with sliced avocado.

Baked Eggs with Parmesan Cheese

Ingredients *(serves 2):*

- 4 large eggs
- 4 tablespoons grated Parmesan cheese (high quality)
- Salt and pepper to taste
- Dried sofrito seasoning

Instructions:

1. Preheat the oven to 350°F (180°C).
2. Place the eggs in a small oven-safe dish.
3. Sprinkle the Parmesan cheese on top and bake for 12-15 minutes.
4. Carefully remove from the oven and sprinkle with dried sofrito for extra flavor.

Low-Carb Bagels

Ingredients:

- 2 cups almond flour
- 1 tablespoon baking powder
- ¼ teaspoon garlic powder *(optional, for a savory flavor)*
- 2½ cups shredded mozzarella cheese
- 2 oz cream cheese
- 2 large eggs
- Sesame seeds, poppy seeds, Everything Bagel seasoning, or cranberry seeds *(optional)*

Instructions:

1. Preheat the oven to 375°F (190°C) and line a baking sheet with parchment paper.
2. In a bowl, combine the almond flour, baking powder, and garlic powder (optional).
3. In a microwave-safe bowl, mix the mozzarella cheese and cream cheese. Microwave in 30-second intervals until fully melted and well combined.
4. Add the eggs to the melted cheese mixture, whisking quickly so the eggs don't cook. Then stir in the dry ingredients and mix until a smooth dough forms.
5. Divide the dough into 6 portions. Roll each into a ball and poke a hole in the center with your fingers to shape it like a bagel. Place on the prepared baking sheet.
6. Optionally, sprinkle seeds or seasoning on top of the bagels before baking.
7. Bake for 12-15 minutes, or until golden brown and firm to the touch.

Optional: Brush with beaten egg before adding toppings for a shinier, golden finish.

Bagel with Smoked Salmon and Cream Cheese

Ingredients *(serves 2):*

- 2 bagels
- 4 oz smoked salmon
- 4 tablespoons cream cheese, at room temperature
- 1 tablespoon aioli

Instructions:

1. Toast the keto bagels.
2. Spread cream cheese on each half and top with smoked salmon.
3. Serve with a side of aioli sauce.

Homemade Aioli Sauce

Makes 1 cup

Ingredients:

- 1 egg
- 1 small garlic clove
- 1 cup olive oil
- 1 tablespoon lemon juice
- Salt to taste

Instructions:

1. In a tall container, add the egg, garlic, lemon juice, and salt.
2. Gently pour in the olive oil on top–do not stir.
3. Using an immersion blender, blend from the bottom of the container for 10 seconds without moving. Then slowly lift the blender to emulsify until the mixture becomes creamy.
4. Transfer the sauce to a container with a lid and spread it on your bagel with salmon.

Avocado, Egg & Cheese Bowl

Ingredients *(serves 2):*

- 1 avocado, halved
- 4 eggs
- ¼ cup spinach
- ¼ cup mushrooms
- ½ cup shredded cheese
- Fresh strawberries

Instructions:

1. In a skillet, add a bit of butter and sauté the spinach and mushrooms until soft, about 3-4 minutes.
2. Add the beaten eggs, seasoned with salt and pepper, and stir until scrambled to your desired doneness.
3. Serve in a bowl: spoon in the scrambled eggs, sprinkle with shredded cheese, and place the sliced avocado and strawberries to the side.
4. Enjoy with a handful of almonds or walnuts.

Almond Flour Crepes with Berries

Ingredients *(makes 2 crepes):*

- 2 large eggs
- 2 tablespoons almond flour
- ¼ teaspoon xanthan gum
- ¼ cup mixed berries
- *Optional:* sugar-free sweetener or date sugar

Instructions:

1. In a bowl, whisk together the eggs, almond flour, and xanthan gum until smooth.
2. Cook small portions in a non-stick skillet over medium heat, spreading the batter thinly.
3. Fill with berries and serve.

Low-Carb Huevos Rancheros

Ingredients *(serves 2):*

- 2 fried eggs
- ¼ cup diced ham
- 2 tablespoons keto-friendly salsa *(see next recipe)*
- 1 tablespoon shredded cheese
- 2 romaine lettuce leaves

Instructions:

1. In a skillet over medium heat, fry the eggs to your desired doneness.
2. Rinse the romaine leaves with cold water and let them rest in ice water for a few minutes to make them extra crisp.
3. Place each fried egg on a lettuce leaf.
4. Top with salsa, diced ham, and shredded cheese.

Ranchera Sauce (Keto-Friendly)

Ingredients:

- 4 large tomatoes or 6 small ones
- 1 jalapeño or serrano pepper
- ¼ white onion
- 2 garlic cloves
- ½ cup chicken broth or water
- 2 tablespoons olive oil or lard
- ½ teaspoon ground cumin
- ½ teaspoon dried oregano
- Salt and pepper to taste
- Fresh cilantro for garnish *(optional)*

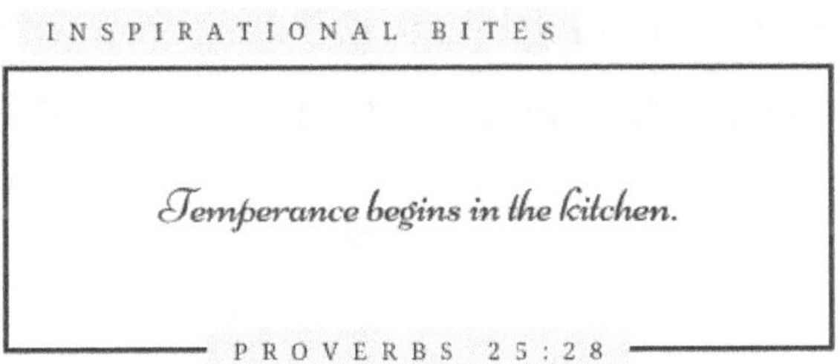

Instructions:

1. Place the tomatoes, pepper, onion, and garlic cloves on a hot skillet or grill (without oil). Roast them until slightly charred on the outside and tender on the inside.
2. In a blender, combine the roasted tomatoes, pepper, onion, garlic, chicken broth, cumin, oregano, salt, and pepper. Blend until smooth or leave it slightly chunky if you prefer a rustic texture.
3. In a skillet, heat the lard or olive oil. Pour in the blended sauce and cook over medium heat for 5-7 minutes, stirring occasionally, until it thickens slightly.
4. Taste and adjust seasoning with more salt and pepper if needed.
5. Garnish with fresh cilantro, if desired, and serve hot over eggs, meat, chicken, or any keto-friendly dish.

Chocolate Walnut Mug Muffin

Ingredients: *(Makes 2 muffins)*

- 4 tablespoons almond flour
- 2 tablespoons unsweetened cocoa powder
- 2 teaspoons chopped walnuts
- 2 small eggs

Instructions:

1. Toast the chopped walnuts in a skillet over medium-high heat to enhance their flavor.
2. Mix all the ingredients in a microwave-safe bowl or mug.
3. Microwave for 1-2 minutes, or until set.
4. Serve with fresh fruit and extra walnuts on top.

Texas-Style Scramble

Ingredients *(Serves 2):*

- 4 large eggs
- ¼ cup unsweetened almond milk *(optional, for extra fluffiness)*
- ½ cup finely chopped red onion
- ½ cup chopped green and red bell peppers
- 1 jalapeño, finely chopped *(optional)*
- ½ cup chopped fresh spinach
- ½ cup diced avocado *(for serving)*
- ½ cup sugar-free chorizo, diced
- ½ cup shredded cheddar cheese
- Salt and pepper to taste
- 1 tablespoon olive oil or ghee butter

Instructions:

1. In a bowl, whisk the eggs with the almond milk (if using), salt, and pepper.
2. In a large skillet, melt the ghee or add olive oil over medium heat.
3. Add the onion and bell peppers. Sauté until tender.
4. Stir in the spinach and chorizo. Cook for an additional 2-3 minutes.
5. Reduce heat to low and pour the beaten eggs over the vegetables.
6. Cook slowly, stirring gently with a spatula until the eggs are nearly set.
7. Add the cheddar cheese and stir until melted.
8. Serve hot, topped with diced avocado.

LUNCHES WITH PURPOSE

Satisfy your body. Ignite your mind.

Lunches

Less sugar at midday. More focus for the rest of the day.

Lunch is that turning point between what you've already accomplished and what's still ahead. Choosing low-carb lunches isn't just a dietary decision–it's a conscious strategy to keep your mind clear, your body active, and your focus sharp throughout the afternoon.

Reducing sugar at midday helps prevent the classic afternoon slump, sudden cravings, and that mental heaviness that often pulls us away from our purpose. Eating with intention during this time of day improves not only your metabolism, but also your decision-making, productivity, and overall well-being.

Here are 10 powerful reasons to make lunch a moment of focus and real nourishment:

1. Stabilizes blood sugar levels
2. Enhances satiety and appetite control
3. Supports weight loss or maintenance
4. Promotes healthy digestion
5. Increases sustained energy
6. Supports brain health and mental clarity

7. Reduces inflammation

8. Helps manage triglycerides and improve heart health

9. Prevents emotional and physical fatigue in the afternoon

10. Fosters a more mindful relationship with food

Having a low-sugar lunch is a simple way to reconnect with yourself–and with what truly matters. In this section, you'll find recipes that not only nourish your body... but also bring your focus back to life.

Chicken Caesar Salad (No Croutons)

Ingredients *(serves 2)*:

- 2 grilled or baked chicken breasts
- 2 cups chopped romaine lettuce
- 2 tablespoons low-carb Caesar dressing
- 2 tablespoons grated Parmesan cheese

Instructions:

1. Season the chicken breasts to your liking.
2. Cook the chicken in a skillet, on the grill, or in the oven.
3. Place the chopped romaine lettuce on a plate.
4. Cut the chicken into bite-sized pieces.
5. Add the chicken, Parmesan cheese, and Caesar dressing to the salad.
6. Toss well and serve.

Note: Swap croutons for pork rinds for a crunchy, low-carb twist.

Lettuce Tacos with Ground Beef

Ingredients *(Makes 2 tacos)*:

- 4 oz lean ground beef, cooked and seasoned with taco spices
- 2 large romaine lettuce leaves
- 2 tablespoons shredded cheese
- 2 tablespoons guacamole
- Sour cream *(optional)*

Instructions:

1. Cook the ground beef to your desired doneness.
2. Season the meat with taco seasoning.
3. Fill each lettuce leaf with the ground beef.
4. Top with shredded cheese, guacamole, and sour cream if desired.
5. Serve immediately.

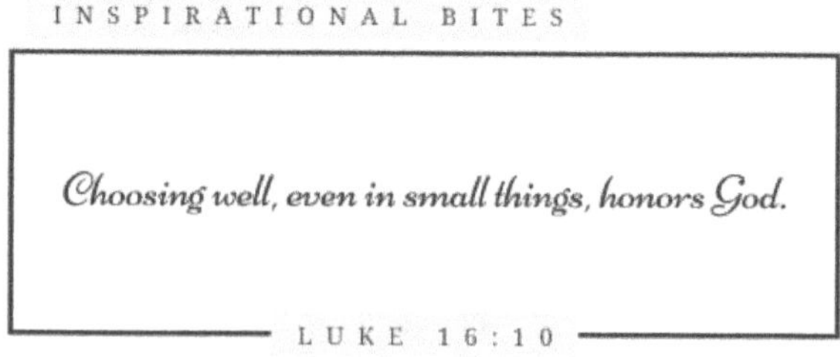

Taco Seasoning (Makes about 8 oz)

Ingredients:

- 1 teaspoon chili powder
- 1 teaspoon ground cumin
- ½ teaspoon paprika
- ¼ teaspoon onion powder
- ¼ teaspoon garlic powder
- ¼ teaspoon dried oregano
- 1/8 teaspoon cayenne pepper *(optional, for heat)*
- Salt and pepper to taste

Instructions:

1. Mix all the ingredients in a bowl. Use immediately and store the rest in an airtight container for future use.

Grilled Chicken Breast with Steamed Broccoli

Ingredients *(serves 2)*:

- 2 chicken breasts
- 2 cups fresh broccoli
- 2 tablespoons olive oil
- Salt and pepper to taste
- Dried sofrito seasoning

Instructions:

1. Season the chicken breasts and grill or bake until golden and cooked through (internal temperature should reach 165°F / 74°C).
2. Steam the broccoli until tender.
3. Serve the chicken with the broccoli and drizzle with olive oil.
4. Sprinkle with dried sofrito for extra flavor.

Pan-Seared Salmon with Asparagus

Ingredients *(serves 2)*:

- 2 skinless salmon fillets
- 12 fresh asparagus spears
- 2 tablespoons butter
- Salt and pepper to taste
- Garlic, to taste
- Lemon juice and zest (separated)
- Dried sofrito seasoning, for garnish

Instructions:

1. Marinate the salmon with garlic, salt, pepper, and lemon juice for about 30 minutes.
2. In a skillet over medium heat, cook the salmon in butter until golden and cooked through.
3. In the same skillet, sauté the asparagus using the flavorful marinade and remaining butter.
4. Serve the salmon with the asparagus.
5. Squeeze a little fresh lemon juice over the top.
6. Garnish with lemon slices, dried sofrito, and lemon zest.

Lettuce-Wrapped Burger

Ingredients:

- 6 oz ground meat *(beef or beef-pork blend)*
- 1 tablespoon avocado mayo
- 1 teaspoon Dijon mustard
- ½ teaspoon garlic powder
- ½ teaspoon onion powder
- Salt and pepper to taste
- 1 tablespoon butter or avocado oil *(for cooking)*

To assemble the burger:

- 2 large lettuce leaves *(iceberg or romaine)*
- 2 tomato slices
- 2 pickle slices
- 1 slice of cheddar cheese *(or your favorite cheese)*
- 1 tablespoon avocado mayo
- 1 fried egg or sliced avocado *(optional)*

Instructions:

1. In a bowl, mix the ground meat with avocado mayo, mustard, garlic powder, onion powder, salt, and pepper. Shape into a burger patty.
2. Heat a skillet with butter over medium-high heat.
3. Cook the burger for 3-4 minutes on each side, or until it reaches your desired doneness. Add the cheese on top and let it melt.
4. Use the lettuce leaves as a substitute for the bun.
5. Place the cheeseburger inside the lettuce wrap and add tomato, pickles, and your favorite condiments.
6. For extra flavor and healthy fats, add a fried egg or avocado slices if desired.
7. Secure the burger with a toothpick.
8. Serve with keto cheese chips and fresh berries.

Lettuce Wraps with Chicken and Avocado

Ingredients *(Serves 4)*:

- 8 large romaine lettuce leaves *(1g net carbs each)*
- 2 chicken breasts, sliced into strips *(or thighs, if preferred)*
- ½ teaspoon garlic powder
- ½ teaspoon dried oregano
- ½ teaspoon ground cumin
- Salt and pepper to taste
- ½ cup fresh spinach
- ¼ cup crumbled truffle cheddar cheese
- Kalamata olives *(optional)*
- 2 tablespoons sun-dried tomatoes
- 1 lemon *(juice used in two separate steps)*
- ½ cup plain, unsweetened Greek yogurt
- Dried dill to taste
- Avocado

Instructions:

1. In a bowl, mix the spinach, cheese, olives, sun-dried tomatoes, 1 tablespoon of lemon juice, and some lemon zest.
2. Slice the chicken breasts into strips and season with garlic powder, oregano, cumin, salt, and pepper.
3. In a skillet over medium-high heat, cook the chicken strips until golden and fully cooked, about 3-4 minutes per side depending on thickness.
4. In a separate bowl, mix the Greek yogurt with 1 tablespoon of lemon juice, garlic, dill, salt, and pepper to make the dressing.
5. Lay out two lettuce leaves per wrap, add chicken and a spoonful of the spinach mixture, and roll the lettuce like a wrap.
6. Cut in half and drizzle with the yogurt sauce. Serve with avocado slices. You can also sprinkle Everything Bagel seasoning on top if desired.

Baked Red Snapper with Cauliflower Mash

Ingredients *(serves 2)*:

- 2 red snapper fillets
- Fresh garlic, to taste
- Salt and pepper
- Extra virgin olive oil
- 2 tablespoons chopped fresh cilantro
- 1 lemon *(both juice and zest)*
- 2 cups steamed cauliflower
- 2 tablespoons ricotta cheese or plain Greek yogurt
- 2 tablespoons butter

Instructions:

1. In a bowl, combine garlic, olive oil, salt, pepper, cilantro, and lemon juice. Marinate the fish fillets in the mixture for about 30 minutes in the refrigerator.
2. Bake the red snapper at 350°F (180°C) for 20-25 minutes, depending on the thickness.
3. In a food processor, blend the steamed cauliflower with ricotta cheese and butter until smooth and creamy.
4. Serve the cauliflower mash with the baked fish on top. Garnish with lemon zest to enhance the flavor.

Note: You can add avocado sauce for a boost of healthy fats.

Greek Salad with Feta Cheese

Ingredients *(Serves 2):*

- 2 cups romaine lettuce
- 1 cup feta cheese
- ½ cucumber, sliced
- Black olives
- Sliced onion
- Toasted walnuts, chopped
- 4 tablespoons plain Greek yogurt
- 2 teaspoons lemon juice
- Salt and pepper to taste
- 1 teaspoon sumac *(or to taste)*

Instructions:

1. In a bowl, combine the lettuce, feta cheese, cucumber, onion slices, olives, and chopped walnuts.
2. In a separate bowl, mix the Greek yogurt, lemon juice, and sumac. Season with salt and pepper to taste.
3. Add the dressing to the salad and toss well.
4. Serve with your favorite protein.

Curry Chicken with Cauliflower Rice

Ingredients *(serves 2)*:

- 16 oz chicken, cubed
- 2 tablespoons low-carb curry paste
- 1 tablespoon sesame oil
- 2 cups cauliflower rice
- ¼ cup red onion, chopped
- ¼ teaspoon grated ginger
- 1 garlic clove, grated
- 1 tablespoon coconut aminos
- Green onions (for garnish)
- 2 scrambled eggs

Instructions:

1. In a skillet, cook the chicken with the curry paste until fully cooked and coated.
2. In another skillet, heat the sesame oil and sauté the red onion with ginger and garlic for 1-2 minutes.
3. Add the cauliflower rice and stir to combine well.
4. Pour in the coconut aminos and mix until everything is evenly coated.
5. Stir in the scrambled eggs.
6. Serve the curry chicken on top of the cauliflower rice.
7. Garnish with chopped green onions.

Stuffed Zucchini with Meat and Cheese

Ingredients *(serves 2)*:

- 2 medium zucchinis
- 1 pound ground meat
- 1 tablespoon sofrito
- Salt and pepper to taste
- 1 teaspoon ground cumin
- 1 teaspoon paprika
- 1 teaspoon turmeric
- Dried oregano to taste *(optional)*
- 2 tablespoons shredded mozzarella cheese

Instructions:

1. Preheat the oven to 350°F (180°C).
2. Slice the zucchinis lengthwise and scoop out a bit of the flesh to create space for filling.
3. In a medium skillet, sauté the sofrito, cumin, paprika, turmeric, and oregano. *(Tip: Rub the oregano between your fingers before adding to intensify the flavor.)*
4. Add the ground meat and cook thoroughly.
5. Fill the zucchini halves with the cooked meat and top with mozzarella cheese.
6. Bake for 15 minutes.

Cabbage Wrap with Turkey and Mustard

Ingredients *(serves 2):*

- 2 large cabbage leaves
- 6 oz cooked turkey, sliced
- Gouda cheese
- 1 tablespoon Dijon mustard
- ½ cup strawberries
- ¼ cup almonds

Instructions:

1. Lay out the cabbage leaves and place the turkey and Gouda cheese in the center.
2. Spread the Dijon mustard, roll up, and serve with strawberries and almonds on the side.

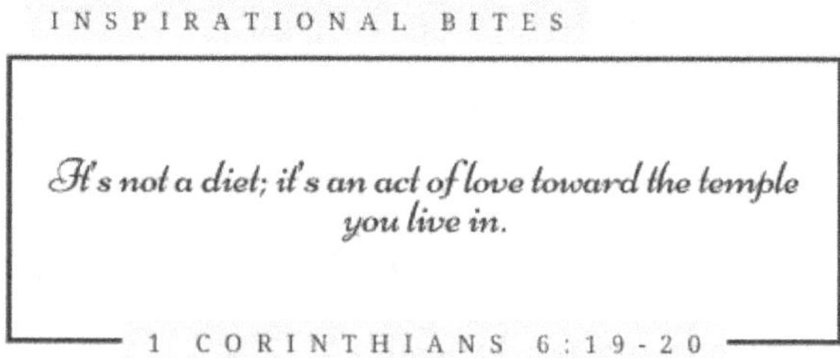

Roasted Turkey Breast with Avocado Salad

Ingredients *(serves 2)*:

- ½ roasted turkey breast
- Salt and pepper
- Olive oil
- 1 sprig of thyme
- ½ avocado, diced
- 1 cup mixed lettuce
- ½ cup cherry tomatoes, halved
- 2 tablespoons olive oil
- 1 tablespoon lemon juice
- Salt and pepper
- Cayenne pepper, to taste

Instructions:

1. Preheat the oven to 350°F (180°C).
2. Slice the turkey breast in half to speed up cooking. Season with salt, pepper, a drizzle of olive oil or butter, and top with thyme.
3. Place on a baking tray and roast for about 30 minutes, flipping halfway through. Make sure the internal temperature reaches 165°F (74°C).
4. In a small bowl, whisk together the olive oil, lemon juice, salt, pepper, and cayenne pepper until emulsified.
5. In a large bowl, combine the lettuce and avocado.
6. To serve, place the salad on a plate, drizzle with the dressing, and top with the turkey breast sliced into strips.

Broccoli and Cheese Soup

Ingredients *(serves 2)*:

- 4 strips of bacon, cut into small pieces
- 2 cups chopped broccoli
- 2 cups low-carb chicken broth
- ¼ cup shredded cheddar cheese
- 1 avocado

Instructions:

1. Cook the bacon pieces until crispy, then remove and set aside.
2. Add the broccoli to the broth and cook until tender. Reserve a small piece for garnish.
3. Blend the soup until smooth, then stir in the cheddar cheese.
4. Simmer on low heat until the cheese is fully melted.
5. Serve in a bowl and garnish with crispy bacon, a bit of the reserved broccoli, and extra cheese if desired.
6. Serve with sliced avocado on the side.

Meatballs in Tomato Sauce

Ingredients *(serves 4):*

- 1 lb ground beef *(or your preferred ground meat)*
- 4 tablespoons almond flour
- 1 beaten egg
- ½ cup no-sugar-added tomato sauce
- Seasonings to taste
- Zucchini noodles (zoodles)
- Grated Parmesan cheese

Instructions:

1. In a bowl, mix the ground meat with almond flour and the beaten egg. Form into meatballs.
2. Cook the meatballs in a skillet until golden browned, then add the tomato sauce.
3. Simmer on low heat for 10 minutes.
4. Add the zucchini noodles, mix well, and serve.
5. Garnish with grated Parmesan cheese and Italian seasoning.

Pork Chops with Sautéed Spinach and Mushrooms

Ingredients *(serves 2)*:

- 4 pork chops, seasoned to your taste
- 4 cups fresh spinach
- 4 sliced mushrooms
- 1 tablespoon olive oil
- 1 avocado

Instructions:

1. Cook the pork chops on the grill, in a skillet, or in an air fryer until golden and the internal temperature reaches 165°F (74°C).
2. Slice the avocado.
3. In a skillet, sauté the spinach and mushrooms in olive oil for 2-3 minutes until tender.
4. Serve the sautéed vegetables as a side with the pork chops.

Grilled Chicken with Arugula Salad

Ingredients *(serves 2)*:

- 2 chicken breasts
- 1 tablespoon olive oil
- ½ tablespoon paprika
- ½ teaspoon garlic powder
- ½ teaspoon onion powder
- ½ teaspoon lemon juice
- Oregano to taste
- Salt and pepper to taste
- 2 cups fresh arugula
- 2 tablespoons lemon and olive oil dressing
- Everything Bagel seasoning

Instructions:

1. In a bowl, mix the olive oil, lemon juice, oregano, paprika, garlic powder, onion powder, salt, and pepper.
2. Marinate the chicken in the mixture for about 10 minutes.
3. Grill or pan-sear the chicken until fully cooked and golden brown.
4. Serve the chicken over the fresh arugula and drizzle with the dressing.
5. Sprinkle with Everything Bagel seasoning.

Homemade Cauliflower Crust Pizza

Ingredients *(serves 2):*

- 1 cauliflower pizza crust
- ¼ cup no-sugar-added tomato sauce
- ¼ cup shredded mozzarella cheese
- Ham
- Pepperoni
- Bacon
- Fresh basil

Instructions:

1. Spread the tomato sauce and cheese over the cauliflower crust. Top with your preferred ingredients: ham, pepperoni, bacon, etc.
2. Bake at 400°F (200°C) for 10-15 minutes until the cheese is melted and bubbly.

Super Easy Cauliflower Pizza Crust

Ingredients:

- 1 medium cauliflower (about 3 cups grated)
- 1 egg
- ½ cup shredded mozzarella cheese
- 2 tablespoons grated Parmesan cheese *(optional, for more flavor)*
- ½ teaspoon salt
- ½ teaspoon garlic powder *(optional)*
- ½ teaspoon dried oregano

Instructions:

1. Preheat your oven to 400°F (200°C) and line a baking sheet with parchment paper.
2. Grate the cauliflower or pulse it in a food processor until it resembles rice.
3. Steam or microwave the cauliflower rice for 3-5 minutes until tender. Let it cool slightly, then place it in a clean kitchen towel and squeeze out as much moisture as possible.
4. In a bowl, mix the cauliflower with the egg, mozzarella, Parmesan, salt, garlic powder, and oregano until a dough forms.
5. Press the dough onto the baking sheet in a circular shape, about ¼ inch thick.
6. Bake for 20-25 minutes or until golden and firm.
7. Add your favorite toppings and return to the oven for another 10-15 minutes until the cheese is bubbly and melted.

Tuna Salad with Hard-Boiled Egg

Ingredients *(serves 2)*:

- 2 cans of tuna in water, drained
- 2 hard-boiled eggs, chopped
- 2 tablespoons low-carb mayonnaise
- 2 cups mixed lettuce greens

Instructions:

1. In a bowl, mix the tuna, chopped eggs, and mayonnaise until well combined.
2. Serve over the bed of mixed greens.

Optional: Add a touch of mustard or diced celery for extra crunch and flavor.

Crab Salmorejo with Cauliflower Rice

Ingredients *(serves 2)*:

- 1 package of cauliflower rice
- 8 oz of crab meat
- 1 chayote, grated
- 2 garlic cloves, minced
- Bell pepper and onion, to taste
- 1 tablespoon sofrito
- 1 tablespoon tomato sauce
- Salt and pepper to taste
- 1 avocado

Instructions:

1. Steam the cauliflower rice and set aside.
2. In a skillet, sauté the bell pepper, onion, garlic, sofrito, and tomato sauce for about 2 minutes.
3. Add the grated chayote and stir to combine.
4. Mix in the crab meat and cook until fully warmed and well blended.
5. Serve the salmorejo over the cauliflower rice and garnish with sliced avocado.

Egg and Bacon Wrap

Ingredients *(Makes 1 wrap)*:

- 1 keto egglife tortilla
- 1 egg
- 1 tablespoon ricotta cheese or cream cheese
- Salt and pepper to taste
- 2 strips of crispy bacon
- Gouda cheese

Instructions:

1. In a skillet, cook the bacon until crispy, then set aside.
2. In a bowl, whisk the egg with the ricotta cheese, salt, and pepper.
3. Cook the egg mixture in a skillet over medium heat. Once cooked, place a bit of Gouda cheese on top and cover until melted.
4. Place the egg and bacon onto the keto egglife tortilla.
5. Roll up the wrap and serve warm.
6. Optional: Serve with fresh berries like strawberries, blueberries, and a few nuts.

Spinach and Cream Cheese Soup

Ingredients *(serves 2)*:

- 2 cups fresh spinach
- 2 cups low-carb chicken broth
- 2 tablespoons cream cheese
- 1 tablespoon heavy cream
- Bacon (optional)
- Shredded cheddar cheese
- Avocado (optional but recommended)

Instructions:

1. In a medium saucepan, cook the spinach in the broth until tender.
2. Add the cream cheese and heavy cream, stirring well to combine.
3. Blend the mixture until smooth and creamy.
4. Return to the saucepan to adjust the consistency, if needed.
5. Serve and garnish with crispy bacon and shredded cheese.
6. Optional: Serve with sliced avocado for extra creaminess and healthy fats.

Beef Steak with Avocado

Ingredients *(serves 2)*:

- 1 lb of your favorite beef steak (avoid pre-cut "steak" strips)
- ½ cup extra virgin olive oil
- ½ cup apple cider vinegar
- Salt and pepper to taste
- ½ onion, thinly sliced
- 2 garlic cloves, minced
- Avocado
- Fresh cilantro for garnish

Instructions:

1. In a bowl, combine the olive oil, minced garlic, and apple cider vinegar.
2. Season the steaks with salt and pepper, then place them in the bowl with the marinade. Let marinate for about 30 minutes.
3. In a skillet, heat olive oil and sear the steaks for about 5 minutes on each side, or until browned.
4. Add the sliced onions to the skillet and mix well to infuse the flavors.
5. Serve with fresh avocado slices.
6. Garnish with chopped cilantro.

Shredded Pork with Sautéed Cabbage

Ingredients *(serves 2)*:

- 1 lb of pork
- 2 garlic cloves
- 1 tablespoon sofrito
- ½ onion, chopped
- 1 teaspoon ground cumin
- 1 teaspoon smoked paprika
- 1 teaspoon parsley
- 1 bay leaf
- 1 cup shredded cabbage
- 1 tablespoon olive oil
- Avocado, for serving

Instructions:

1. In a saucepan over medium heat, cook the pork for about 30 minutes with garlic, bay leaf, onion, sofrito, and salt, until the meat is tender and easy to shred with a fork.
2. In a skillet, sauté the cabbage in olive oil until tender.
3. Add the shredded pork and mix well until combined.
4. Serve with a slice of fresh avocado.

Baked Cauliflower Casserole

Ingredients *(serves 2)*:

- 1 fresh cauliflower
- ½ cup diced ham
- ½ cup shredded cheese

Instructions:

1. Wash and cut the cauliflower into small pieces.
2. Steam the cauliflower until tender.
3. Lightly butter a baking dish and add the cooked cauliflower and diced ham.
4. Sprinkle with shredded cheese and bake at 350°F (180°C) for 15 minutes or until the cheese is melted and golden brown.

Zucchini Roll-Ups with Ground Meat

Ingredients *(serves 2)*:

- 2 zucchinis
- 1 lb ground meat (your choice)
- ¼ green bell pepper
- ¼ onion
- 2 tablespoons sofrito
- Salt and pepper to taste
- Paprika
- Oregano
- Basil
- 4 Baby Bella mushrooms, sliced
- ½ cup sugar-free tomato sauce
- Mozzarella cheese
- Parmesan cheese

Instructions:

1. Wash and slice the zucchinis into very thin strips using a vegetable peeler for uniform slices. Place the slices on a paper towel to absorb excess moisture.
2. In a skillet, add olive oil, chopped onion and pepper, garlic paste, a bit of tomato sauce, and the sofrito. Sauté until it forms a fragrant paste.
3. Add the ground meat and cook until fully done. Let the mixture cool.
4. In an oven-safe dish, spread a thin layer of tomato sauce on the bottom.
5. Take 2 slices of zucchini, add some of the ground meat mixture, and roll them up to form a roll-up. Place each roll in the dish.
6. Once all roll-ups are in the dish, top with more tomato sauce and your desired amount of mozzarella and parmesan cheese.
7. Bake at 350°F (180°C) for about 15 minutes.
8. Garnish with finely chopped cilantro or basil.

Chicken Bowl with Avocado, Spinach & Lemon Dressing

Ingredients *(serves 2)*:

- 2 chicken breasts
- Salt and pepper
- ½ avocado
- 2 cups fresh spinach
- ¼ cup fresh lemon juice
- ½ cup extra virgin olive oil
- 1 garlic clove, grated
- 1 teaspoon Dijon mustard
- Salt and pepper to taste
- Lemon zest

Instructions:

1. Season the chicken breasts with salt and pepper, then grill or pan-sear until fully cooked (165°F internal temp). Let rest a few minutes before slicing into cubes.
2. In a small bowl, whisk together the lemon juice, olive oil, grated garlic, Dijon mustard, and lemon zest until emulsified. Adjust salt and pepper to taste.
3. In a bowl or plate, arrange the spinach and top with the cubed chicken.
4. Drizzle with the lemon dressing and garnish with more lemon zest and sliced avocado.

Chicken Breasts in Creamy Mushroom Sauce

Ingredients *(serves 2):*

- 2 chicken breasts
- Salt and pepper
- Paprika
- ½ cup butter
- 1 lb mushrooms
- 2 garlic cloves
- ¼ cup white wine
- ½ cup chicken broth
- 1 cup heavy cream
- ½ cup grated Parmesan cheese
- 1 avocado

Instructions:

1. Season the chicken breasts with salt, pepper, and paprika.
2. In a skillet, sear the chicken breasts in half of the butter until golden on both sides. Transfer to the oven and finish cooking at 350°F until the internal temperature reaches 165°F.
3. In the same skillet, add the remaining butter and sauté the mushrooms and garlic for about 3 minutes.
4. Add the white wine and deglaze the pan, reducing by half.
5. Pour in the chicken broth. Once it begins to boil, add the heavy cream and Parmesan cheese. Stir until the sauce thickens and becomes creamy.
6. Adjust seasoning with salt and pepper. (Optional: Add a pinch of nutmeg for a deeper flavor.)
7. Return the chicken breasts to the skillet and coat them well with the sauce.
8. Garnish with chopped chives and serve with sliced avocado.

Grilled Pork and Vegetable Skewers

Ingredients *(serves 2)*:

- 1 lb pork, cut into cubes
- 3 garlic cloves, mashed
- Salt and pepper
- Onion, cut into chunks
- ½ red bell pepper, cut into chunks
- 4 mushrooms
- ½ zucchini, sliced
- 6 wooden skewers

Instructions:

1. Soak the wooden skewers in water to prevent them from burning quickly on the grill.
2. Season the pork with garlic, salt, and pepper.
3. Thread the pork and vegetables onto the skewers in the order you prefer (e.g., pork, onion, bell pepper, mushroom, zucchini).
4. Grill the skewers until the meat is cooked through and the vegetables are tender.
5. Optional: Brush the skewers with garlic butter for extra flavor.
6. Serve with grilled mini bell peppers.

Zucchini Noodles with Alfredo Sauce and Shrimp

Ingredients *(serves 2)*:

- 2 cups spiralized zucchini
- 12 fresh shrimp
- Salt and pepper
- Butter
- 2 oz cream cheese
- ¼ cup heavy cream
- Parmesan cheese
- Garlic powder

Instructions:

1. Clean the shrimp and season with salt, pepper, and paprika.
2. In a skillet over medium heat, melt the butter and cook the shrimp for about 3 minutes on each side until golden. Remove and set aside.
3. In the same skillet, sauté the zucchini noodles for 2-3 minutes.
4. Add the cream cheese, heavy cream, and Parmesan cheese. Stir until creamy.
5. Return the shrimp to the skillet and toss everything together until the shrimp and noodles are well coated in the Alfredo sauce.
6. Serve with avocado and a sprinkle of Parmesan cheese.

Beef Stir-Fry with Broccoli, Cauliflower & Lemon

Ingredients *(serves 2)*:

- 1 lb sirloin beef, thinly sliced
- 1 cup broccoli florets
- 1 cup cauliflower florets
- 2 tablespoons olive oil
- 2 garlic cloves, minced
- 1 teaspoon fresh grated ginger
- Juice of 1 large lemon
- Lemon zest
- 2 tablespoons coconut aminos
- 1 teaspoon toasted sesame oil
- Salt and pepper to taste
- Toasted sesame seeds for garnish

Instructions:

1. Marinate the beef with lemon juice, coconut aminos, garlic, ginger, and pepper for 15 to 30 minutes.
2. Heat olive oil in a large skillet or wok over high heat.
3. Stir-fry the beef until browned, then remove and set aside.
4. In the same skillet, stir-fry the broccoli and cauliflower until al dente. Add more oil if needed.
5. Return the beef to the skillet, toss everything together, and adjust salt and lemon to taste.
6. Finish with toasted sesame oil and sprinkle with sesame seeds if desired.
7. Serve with cauliflower rice and avocado.

DINNERS THAT RESTORE

Light on the plate. Deep in rest.

Less Sugar at Night.

More Rest, Clarity, and Wellbeing.

Eating an early, low-carb dinner isn't just a healthy practice–it's an intentional way to care for your body, your mind, and your rest. Instead of ending the day with a heavy load of sugar and processed foods, choosing a light, balanced meal sets you up for restorative sleep, efficient digestion, and a morning filled with energy and focus.

When we finish the day with less sugar, we give our bodies the chance to restore instead of having to work hard on digestion through the night. This simple shift can completely transform your metabolic health, mental clarity, and overall quality of life.

Here are **8 powerful reasons** to embrace this habit:

1. **Improves sleep quality:** A low-carb dinner allows the body to relax faster, promoting deep and restorative rest.
2. **Stabilizes blood sugar levels:** Avoiding nighttime glucose spikes prevents sleep disruptions and early morning cravings.

3. **Supports weight loss or maintenance:** Eating early gives your body time to digest and use stored fat for energy overnight.
4. **Enhances digestion:** Light dinners reduce acidity and bloating and support a healthier gut microbiome.
5. **Boosts metabolic health:** This habit increases insulin sensitivity and helps prevent diseases like type 2 diabetes.
6. **Promotes nighttime ketosis:** Lower carb intake in the evening helps the body enter ketosis, burning fat for fuel while you sleep.
7. **Reduces inflammation:** Avoiding refined carbs and heavy meals at night lowers inflammatory markers.
8. **Supports intermittent fasting:** If you practice fasting, eating an early and light dinner makes the overnight fast easier and more effective.

A mindful, sugar-conscious dinner is a powerful way to end your day with intention.

Example of a Low-Carb Early Dinner

- **Protein:** Grilled fish fillet or chicken
- **Healthy fat:** A quarter of an avocado or a drizzle of olive oil

- **Vegetables:** Asparagus, sautéed spinach, or a fresh salad

- **Optional:** A light broth or non-starchy vegetable soup

Grilled Salmon with Garlic Asparagus

Ingredients *(serves 2)*:

- 2 salmon fillets
- 12 asparagus spears
- 2 tablespoons olive oil
- 2 cloves garlic, minced
- Salt and pepper to taste

Instructions:

1. Preheat the grill or a skillet. Cook the salmon until golden and fully cooked through.
2. In a separate pan, sauté the asparagus with olive oil and garlic until tender.
3. Serve the salmon with the garlic asparagus on the side.

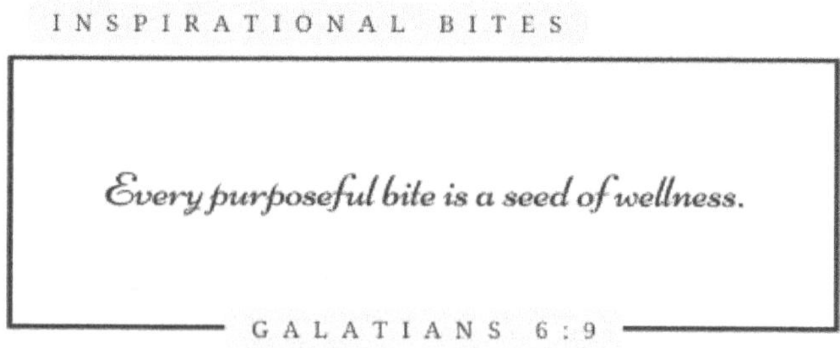

Chicken Breast in Mustard Sauce with Sautéed Kale

Ingredients *(serves 2)*:

- 2 chicken breasts
- 1 tablespoon olive oil
- ½ tablespoon apple cider vinegar
- Salt and pepper to taste
- 2 garlic cloves, mashed into a paste
- Paprika to taste
- 2 cups kale
- 2 tablespoons Dijon mustard
- 1 tablespoon heavy cream
- Fresh cilantro for garnish

Instructions:

1. In a bowl, mix the olive oil, vinegar, garlic paste, paprika, salt, and pepper. Marinate the chicken in the refrigerator for about 30 minutes.
2. Grill or pan-sear the chicken until fully cooked.
3. Mix the Dijon mustard and heavy cream to create the sauce.
4. Sauté the kale until tender and serve it alongside the chicken.
5. Drizzle the mustard sauce over the chicken and garnish with fresh cilantro.

Eggplant Pizza with Cheese and Pepperoni

Ingredients *(serves 2)*:

- 2 medium eggplants, sliced
- 4 tablespoons sugar-free tomato sauce
- ½ cup shredded mozzarella cheese
- 8 slices of pepperoni

Instructions:

1. Slice the eggplants and place them on a tray. Sprinkle salt on both sides and let sit for about 20 minutes to remove bitterness and improve texture–this makes them firmer and less spongy. Then rinse and pat dry.
2. Preheat the oven to 400°F (200°C).
3. Place the eggplant slices on a baking sheet. Add tomato sauce, cheese, and pepperoni on top.
4. Bake for 10-12 minutes or until the cheese is melted and bubbly.

Grilled Beef with Spinach and Avocado Salad

Ingredients *(serves 2)*:

- 1 lb of beef for grilling
- Salt and pepper to taste
- 2 cups fresh spinach
- 1 avocado, sliced
- 2 tablespoons low-carb dressing or vinaigrette

Instructions:

1. Season the beef with salt and pepper.
2. Grill or cook the beef to your preferred doneness.
3. In a bowl, mix the spinach, avocado, and dressing or vinaigrette.
4. Adjust salt if needed.
5. Serve the grilled beef alongside the salad.

Mushroom Basil Cauli-Risotto

Ingredients *(serves 2)*:

- 2 tablespoons of butter or ghee
- ¼ red onion or shallots, finely chopped
- Mushrooms to taste
- 2 garlic cloves, minced
- ¼ cup of white wine
- Fresh basil leaves
- 1 package of riced cauliflower
- Salt and pepper to taste
- 1½ cups of heavy cream
- Pecorino or Parmesan cheese

Instructions:

1. In a skillet, melt the butter until lightly caramelized.
2. Add the onion and cook until translucent.
3. Add the mushrooms and cook until tender.
4. Add the garlic and white wine; cook until the wine reduces by half.
5. Add the fresh basil until aromatic, then stir in the riced cauliflower and mix thoroughly.
6. Add the heavy cream and cheese; stir until it thickens and becomes rich and creamy.

Chicken Sancocho (Hearty Stew)

Ingredients *(serves 2)*:

- 1 grated carrot (optional)
- ½ chopped onion
- ½ green bell pepper
- 1 celery stalk
- 2 garlic cloves
- 1 cup fresh spinach
- 2 chicken thighs with skin and bone
- Salt and pepper to taste
- 1 chayote squash
- 1 rutabaga
- 2 tablespoons sofrito
- 2 bay leaves
- 1 tablespoon olive oil

Instructions:

1. In a medium pot over high heat, cook the chicken thighs with skin on. It's okay if the skin sticks to the bottom–we'll remove it shortly. Remove the chicken and shred it.
2. In the same pot, add onion, bell pepper, carrot, and celery. Sauté until they become translucent.
3. Add sofrito, bay leaves, and olives (optional). Let cook for a few minutes.
4. Peel and chop the chayote and rutabaga into even pieces.
5. Add the chayote and rutabaga to the pot and pour in enough water to cover everything.
6. Shred the chicken and return it to the pot.
7. Season with salt, pepper, and turmeric for color.
8. Simmer until the vegetables are soft, flavors are well combined, and the broth has slightly reduced.
9. Serve with avocado and optional cauliflower rice.

Teriyaki Chicken with Broccoli

Ingredients *(serves 2)*:

- 2 chicken breasts, cut into chunks
- 2 tablespoons low-carb teriyaki sauce
- ½ tablespoon coconut aminos
- 2 cups broccoli florets
- Mini bell peppers

Instructions:

1. Cook the chicken in a skillet with the teriyaki sauce and coconut aminos until fully cooked and glazed.
2. Steam the broccoli until tender but still vibrant.
3. Sauté the mini bell peppers until lightly charred and tender.
4. Serve the chicken with the broccoli and peppers.
5. Garnish with toasted sesame seeds.

Smoked Pork Chops with Broccoli Purée

Ingredients *(serves 2)*:

- 2 smoked pork chops
- Salt and pepper to taste
- 2 cups broccoli florets
- 2 tablespoons heavy cream
- 1 tablespoon pickled onions

Instructions:

1. Cook the pork chops to your desired doneness.
2. Steam the broccoli until tender.
3. Blend the broccoli with the heavy cream to create a purée.
4. If the purée is too runny, simmer it on the stovetop until it thickens.
5. Serve the pork chops with the broccoli purée, and top with pickled onions and a sprinkle of fresh cilantro.

Cheesy Chicken and Mushroom Casserole

Ingredients *(serves 2)*:

- 2 cooked chicken breasts, chopped
- 2 cups mushrooms, sliced
- ½ cup shredded cheese
- 2 tablespoons heavy cream

Instructions:

1. In a casserole dish, combine the chicken, mushrooms, and heavy cream.
2. Sprinkle the shredded cheese on top and bake at 350°F (180°C) for 15 minutes.

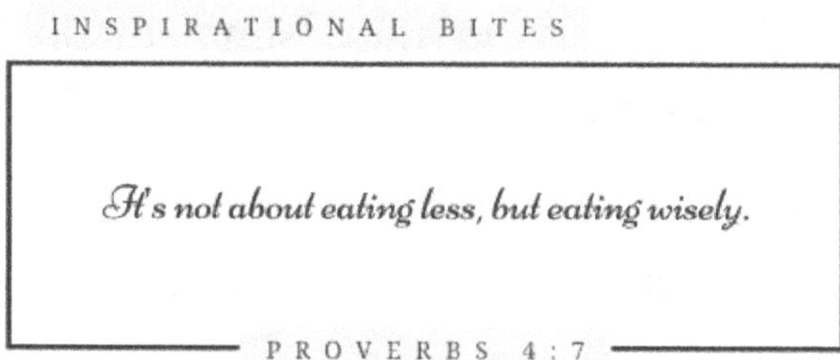

Steamed Fish with Asparagus and Lemon

Ingredients *(serves 2)*:

- 2 hake fillets or your favorite fish
- 12 asparagus spears
- 4 lemon slices
- Salt and pepper to taste

Instructions:

1. Place the fish and asparagus in a steamer basket or steaming dish.
2. Season with salt and pepper and add the lemon slices.
3. Steam for 10-12 minutes.

Cheese Tacos

Ingredients *(for 4 tacos):*

- 2 cups shredded cheese
- ½ cup ground beef or chicken
- Optional: lettuce and keto-friendly salsa

Instructions:

1. Place portions of shredded cheese in a non-stick skillet and cook until golden and crispy.
2. Remove and fold while still warm to form taco shells.
3. Fill with meat and optional toppings.

Baked Chicken with Spinach and Coconut Cream

Ingredients *(serves 2)*:

- 2 chicken breasts
- 2 cups fresh spinach
- ¼ cup unsweetened coconut cream

Instructions:

1. Place the chicken on a baking tray and season with salt and pepper.
2. Bake at 350°F (180°C) for 20-25 minutes.
3. Sauté the spinach in the coconut cream and serve alongside the chicken.

Warm Spinach Salad with Poached Egg

Ingredients *(serves 2)*:

- 4 cups fresh spinach, washed and dried
- 2 poached eggs
- 1 tablespoon vinegar (for poaching the eggs)
- ¼ cup fresh strawberries, chopped
- 2 tablespoons balsamic vinegar
- 1 tablespoon honey
- 1 teaspoon Dijon mustard
- ¼ cup extra virgin olive oil
- 1 very ripe strawberry, mashed (to enhance flavor)
- Walnuts (optional)
- Goat cheese (optional)

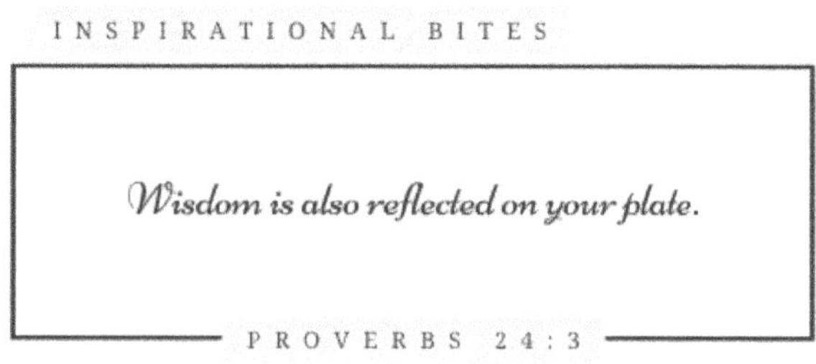

Instructions:

1. Poach the eggs in hot water with vinegar for 3-4 minutes.
2. In a small cup or bowl, whisk together the balsamic vinegar, honey, mustard, olive oil, and mashed strawberry until emulsified.
3. Place the spinach on a plate and top with the poached egg.
4. Add the chopped strawberries, drizzle the vinaigrette over the salad, and sprinkle with walnuts.
5. Crumble goat cheese on top just before serving to preserve its flavor.

Beef Steak with Herb Butter and Cauliflower

Ingredients *(serves 2)*:

- 2 beef steaks of your choice
- 2 cups cooked cauliflower
- 2 tablespoons butter mixed with herbs

Instructions:

1. Cook the steaks to your desired doneness.
2. Serve with cooked cauliflower and drizzle with melted herb butter.

Garlic Shrimp with Steamed Broccoli

Ingredients *(serves 2)*:

- 1 pound shrimp
- 2 tablespoons butter
- 2 tablespoons olive oil
- 1 tablespoon fresh sofrito
- 1 tablespoon young Chardonnay (to enhance the buttery flavor)
- Salt and pepper to taste
- Paprika to taste
- 2 cups steamed broccoli with a pinch of salt
- 1 garlic clove, minced

Instructions:

1. In a skillet over medium-high heat, sauté the sofrito and paprika until fragrant.
2. Add the shrimp and minced garlic to the skillet and cook until the shrimp turn pink, about 2 minutes per side.
3. Pour in the Chardonnay and let it reduce by half.
4. Adjust salt and pepper to taste.
5. Serve with steamed broccoli as a side.
6. Garnish with a pinch of dried sofrito to enhance the flavor.

Chicken Fajitas

Ingredients:

- 1 lb chicken breast, cut into strips
- 1 red bell pepper, sliced
- 1 green bell pepper, sliced
- 1 red onion, sliced
- 2 tablespoons avocado or olive oil
- Juice of 1 lime
- 1 teaspoon ground cumin
- 1 teaspoon paprika
- ½ teaspoon garlic powder
- ½ teaspoon chili powder (optional for heat)
- Salt and pepper to taste
- Fresh cilantro for garnish
- Avocado or guacamole
- Shredded cheese
- Lettuce leaves (to use as "tortillas")
- Lime wedges
- Sugar-free sour cream

Instructions:

1. Marinate the chicken, in a bowl, mix the lime juice, oil, cumin, paprika, garlic powder, salt, pepper, and chili powder. Add the chicken strips and let marinate for 15-30 minutes.
2. Sauté: In a large skillet over medium-high heat, cook the chicken until browned. Remove and set aside.
3. In the same skillet, sauté the peppers and onion until tender-crisp (about 5 minutes).
4. Return the chicken to the skillet and stir everything together for 2 more minutes to blend the flavors.
5. Spoon the mixture onto lettuce leaves and top with avocado, sour cream, or your favorite toppings.

INSPIRATIONAL BITES

God didn't give you a body to punish it, but to serve with it.

ROMANS 12:1

Chicken and Cheese Stuffed Zucchini

Ingredients *(serves 2)*:

• 4 small zucchinis, halved lengthwise

• 2 shredded chicken breasts

• ½ cup of shredded cheese

Instructions:

1. Clean the zucchinis, trim the ends, scoop out the pulp, and fill them with the shredded chicken and cheese.
2. Bake at 350°F (180°C) for 15 minutes or until the cheese is golden.

Burgers with Portobello Buns

Ingredients *(for 2 burgers):*

- 4 large portobello mushrooms
- 2 beef or chicken burger patties
- 1 lettuce leaf and 1 tomato slice
- Provolone cheese
- Low-carb mayonnaise and ketchup
- Avocado
- Caramelized onions

Instructions:

1. Grill the portobello mushrooms until tender.
2. Grill the burger patties until they reach 165°F (74°C).
3. Use the portobellos as buns and fill with the burger patty.
4. Add the lettuce, tomato, cheese, and sauces.
5. Optionally, top with avocado and caramelized onions.

Garlic Salmon with Roasted Brussels Sprouts

Ingredients *(serves 2)*:

- 2 salmon fillets or your favorite fish
- 2 cups Brussels sprouts, halved
- 2 tablespoons olive oil
- Salt and pepper
- 2 garlic cloves, minced
- 1 avocado

Instructions:

1. Roast the Brussels sprouts with olive oil and garlic in the oven at 400°F (200°C) for 20 minutes.
2. Season the fish with salt and pepper, then cook in a skillet with garlic until done.
3. Serve the salmon with the roasted Brussels sprouts and sliced avocado.

Cabbage Rolls with Ground Beef and Keto Sauce

Ingredients *(serves 2)*:

- 4 large cabbage leaves, blanched
- ½ pound ground beef
- ½ cup low-carb tomato sauce
- Parmesan cheese

Instructions:

1. Blanch the cabbage leaves in hot water to soften for rolling.
2. Cook the ground beef to your desired doneness.
3. Fill the cabbage leaves with the cooked beef.
4. Place the rolls in a saucepan, cover with tomato sauce, and sprinkle with Parmesan or your favorite cheese.
5. Cook over low heat for 15 minutes, until the cheese is melted.

Creamy Mushroom and Chicken Soup

Ingredients *(serves 2)*:

- 2 boneless, skinless chicken thighs, chopped into small pieces
- Salt and pepper
- 1 teaspoon sofrito
- 2 cups sliced mushrooms
- 2 cups chicken broth
- 4 tablespoons heavy cream

Instructions:

1. In a hot saucepan, add the chopped chicken with salt and pepper, and mix well.
2. Cook the chicken until it is caramelized and golden brown.
3. Add the mushrooms and sauté them in the broth until tender.
4. Pour in the chicken broth and bring to a boil; let it reduce by half.
5. Add the heavy cream, mix well, and cook for 5 more minutes.
6. Serve with caramelized onions on top.

Baked Salmon with Garlic Butter and Asparagus

Ingredients *(serves 2)*:

- 2 salmon fillets
- 12 asparagus spears
- 2 tablespoons garlic butter

Instructions:

1. On a baking tray lined with parchment paper, place the salmon and asparagus.
2. Drizzle with garlic butter and bake at 350°F (180°C) for 12-15 minutes.
3. Serve and enjoy.

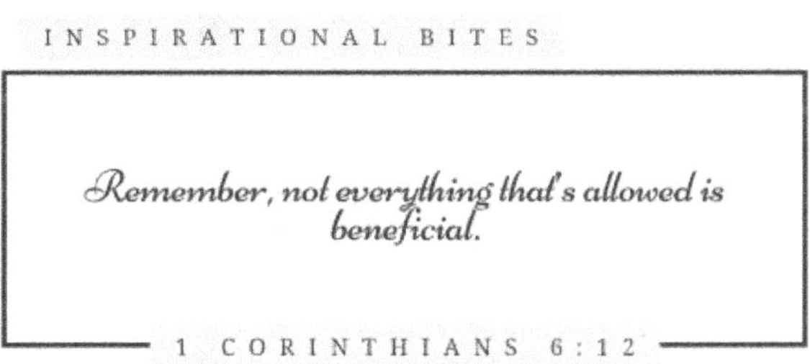

Chicken, Avocado & Kale Bowl

Ingredients *(serves 2)*:

- 4 chicken thighs, chopped (breasts can be used instead)
- 1 avocado, sliced
- 2 cups kale
- 2 tablespoons low-carb dressing
- Everything bagel seasoning to taste

Instructions:

1. Cook the chicken to your liking, preferably grilled.
2. Combine all ingredients in a bowl.
3. Serve cold or warm, depending on your preference.
4. Garnish with everything bagel seasoning to taste.

Curry Chicken with Coconut Cream and Spinach

Ingredients *(serves 2)*:

- 2 chicken breasts, cut into chunks
- 1 cup fresh spinach
- 4 tablespoons coconut cream
- 2 teaspoons curry paste
- Green onions (for garnish)

Instructions:

1. Cut the chicken breasts into evenly sized cubes for even cooking.
2. Cook the chicken with the curry paste until golden.
3. Add the spinach and coconut cream and cook for 5 more minutes.
4. Garnish with chopped green onions.

Shrimp Salad with Roasted Pepper Sauce, Avocado, and Cucumbers

Ingredients *(serves 2)*:

- 1 pound shrimp
- 1 red bell pepper
- 2 garlic cloves
- 2 tablespoons olive oil
- ¼ cup chopped onion
- ½ cup coconut milk or cream (optional)
- ½ avocado
- ½ cucumber, sliced
- Lime juice
- 1 tablespoon additional olive oil

Instructions:

1. Roast the red bell pepper directly over an open flame or in the oven until the skin is blackened. Place it in a covered container for 10 minutes, then peel and remove the seeds.
2. In a skillet, sauté the garlic and onion until golden.
3. Add the roasted pepper and sauté for 1-2 more minutes.
4. Transfer everything to a blender, add the coconut milk or cream, and blend until smooth and creamy.
5. Return the sauce to the skillet, season with salt and pepper.
6. Add the shrimp and a splash of lime juice, and cook until the shrimp are done.
7. In a bowl, combine the avocado and cucumber slices.
8. Add the shrimp in the sauce and toss everything together gently.

Cheesy Baked Eggplant with Ground Beef

Ingredients *(serves 2)*:

- 2 medium eggplants
- Salt
- 1 pound ground beef
- ½ cup shredded cheese

Instructions:

1. Slice the eggplants and place them on a tray lined with paper towels. Sprinkle with salt to remove bitterness and improve texture.
2. Let sit for about 10 minutes, then rinse.
3. Cook the eggplant slices in a skillet until tender.
4. Fill them with cooked ground beef and sprinkle with cheese.
5. Bake at 350°F (180°C) for 10 minutes.

Chicken and Vegetable Skewers

Ingredients *(serves 2)*:

- 2 chicken breasts or 4 chicken thighs, cut into cubes
- Salt and pepper
- Garlic paste
- 1 red bell pepper, cubed
- 1 onion, cubed
- 1 zucchini, sliced
- 4 mushrooms, sliced

Instructions:

1. Cut all ingredients into roughly 2x2 cm cubes.
2. Season the chicken with salt, pepper, and garlic paste.
3. Thread the chicken and vegetables onto skewers.
4. Grill until golden and fully cooked.
5. Serve with grilled vegetables on the side.

Tomato Soup with Parmesan Cheese

Ingredients *(serves 2)*:

- 1 cup unsweetened crushed tomatoes
- 1 cup chicken broth
- 1 tablespoon sofrito
- 2 tablespoons grated Parmesan cheese

Instructions:

1. Cook the tomatoes in the chicken broth with the sofrito until well combined and heated through.
2. Add the Parmesan cheese and stir well before serving.
3. Optional: Make Parmesan crisps for a crunchy topping.
   - Place grated Parmesan in a skillet over medium heat until fully melted and golden.
   - Remove carefully and let cool to crisp up before adding to the soup.

Creamy Chicken with Steamed Broccoli

Ingredients *(serves 2)*:

- 2 chicken breasts, cut into pieces
- Salt and pepper
- 2 cups steamed broccoli
- 4 tablespoons heavy cream

Instructions:

1. Season the chicken with salt and pepper.
2. Cook the chicken in a skillet until golden brown.
3. Add the heavy cream and mix well.
4. Serve with steamed broccoli on the side.

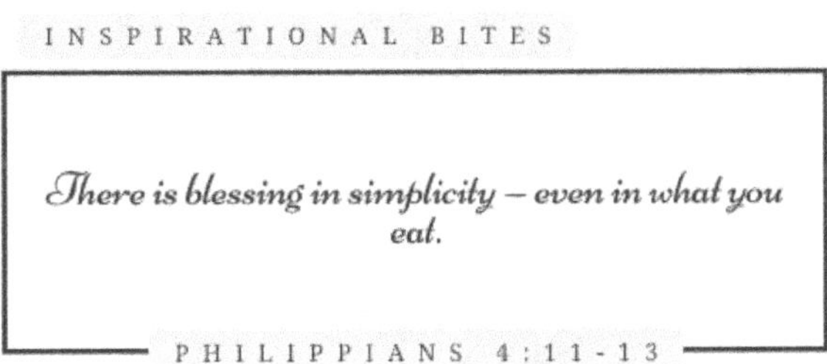

SNACKS WITH INTENTION
Small bites, big decisions

SNACKS WITH INTENTION

Fewer cravings. More focus between meals.

Snack time is often the most vulnerable moment of the day: energy drops, stress rises, and the body–or rather, the mind– craves "something quick." But that "something" doesn't have to be high in sugar or sabotage your goals. Choosing low-carb snacks is a smart and practical way to keep your energy stable, curb emotional hunger, and sustain focus between meals.

A balanced snack not only helps you avoid glucose spikes and crashes, but also fuels your brain with what it really needs to stay sharp–without anxiety, fatigue, or distraction.

Here are 7 reasons to choose low-carb snacks:

1. **They prevent sugar spikes:** By avoiding sugary snacks, you keep glucose levels stable and your mind clear.
2. **They prolong satiety:** Combinations of protein and healthy fats help you reach your next meal without extreme hunger.
3. **They improve mental focus:** Reducing simple sugars helps lower mental fatigue and keeps your concentration steady.
4. **They reduce emotional cravings:** A mindful snack helps you distinguish real hunger from anxiety-driven eating.
5. **They support weight loss or maintenance:** By controlling food impulses, you avoid empty calorie overload.

6. **They promote balanced metabolism:** Low-carb snacks stabilize insulin response between meals.
7. **They align with your purpose:** Eating with intention–even between meals–is a way of honoring your body as a temple.

A snack isn't an excuse to break your routine it's an opportunity to reinforce your commitment to health and focus.

Examples of Low-Carb Snacks
• Ham rolls with cream cheese
• Cucumber slices with low-carb hummus
• Nuts or almonds in a controlled portion
• Boiled eggs
• Celery sticks with natural peanut butter
• Unsweetened Greek yogurt with cinnamon
• Baked cheese chips or cheese slices

Mixed Nuts

Ingredients:

• ¼ cup of unsalted mixed nuts (almonds, walnuts, pecans)

Instructions:

1.   Measure a ¼ cup serving and enjoy as a snack.

Cucumber Slices with Cream Cheese

Ingredients:
• ½ cucumber, sliced
• 2 tablespoons of cream cheese

Instructions:

1.   Spread cream cheese on the cucumber slices and serve.
2.   Garnish with Everything Bagel Seasoning.

Green or Black Olives

Ingredients:

• 10 green or black olives.

Instructions:

1. Serve the olives as a snack.

Ham Rolls with Cream Cheese

Ingredients:

• 2 slices of low-sodium ham
• 2 tablespoons of cream cheese

Instructions:

1. Spread cream cheese on the ham slices and roll them up.

Avocado Chunks with Salt and Lime

Ingredients:

- ½ avocado, cut into chunks
- Salt and lime to taste

Instructions:

1. Season the avocado chunks with salt and lime.

Cheddar Cheese Cubes

Ingredients:

- ¼ cup of cheddar cheese, cubed

Instructions:

1. Cut the cheese into cubes and serve.

Baked Kale Chips

Ingredients:

- 1 cup of kale
- 1 tablespoon of olive oil
- Salt to taste

Instructions:

1. Toss the kale with olive oil and salt.
2. Bake at 350°F (180°C) for 10-15 minutes.

Hard-Boiled Eggs

Ingredients:

- 2 eggs

Instructions:

1. Boil the eggs in water for 10 minutes, peel, and serve.

Cottage Cheese with Strawberries

Ingredients:

- ½ cup of cottage cheese
- 2 chopped strawberries

Instructions:

1. Mix the cottage cheese with the strawberries and serve.

Crispy Cheese Chips

Ingredients:

- ½ cup of shredded cheese

Instructions:

1. Place small piles of shredded cheese on a baking tray and bake at 400°F (200°C) for 5-7 minutes.

Celery Sticks with Natural Peanut Butter

Ingredients:

- 2 celery stalks
- 1 tablespoon of natural peanut butter

Instructions:

1. Spread the peanut butter on the celery sticks and serve.

Smoked Salmon Rolls with Cream Cheese

Ingredients:

- 2 slices of smoked salmon
- 2 tablespoons of cream cheese

Instructions:

1. Spread cream cheese on the salmon slices and roll them up.

Bell Pepper Slices with Keto Hummus

Ingredients:

- ½ bell pepper, sliced
- 2 tablespoons of keto hummus

Instructions:

1. Serve the bell pepper slices with hummus as a dip.

Mini Eggplant Pizza with Cheese

Ingredients:

- 1 eggplant, sliced
- ¼ cup of mozzarella cheese

Instructions:

1. Top the eggplant slices with cheese and bake at 400°F (200°C) for 10 minutes.

Pork Rinds

Ingredients:

• ¼ cup of pork rinds

Instructions:

1. Serve directly as a snack.

Coconut and Almond Butter Energy Balls

Ingredients:

• 2 tablespoons of almond butter
• 2 tablespoons of unsweetened shredded coconut

Instructions:

1. Mix the ingredients, form small balls, and refrigerate for 30 minutes.

Cucumbers with Salt and Vinegar

Ingredients:

- ½ cucumber, sliced
- Vinegar and salt to taste

Instructions:

1. Mix the cucumber slices with vinegar and salt.

Zucchini Chunks with Guacamole

Ingredients:

- 1 zucchini, cut into chunks
- 2 tablespoons of guacamole

Instructions:

1. Serve the zucchini chunks with guacamole as a dip.

Small Avocado and Tomato Salad

Ingredients:

- ½ avocado
- 1 small tomato

Instructions:

1. Mix the avocado and tomato in a bowl and season to taste.

Chicken Rolls with Mozzarella Cheese

Ingredients:

- 2 slices of cooked chicken
- 2 strips of mozzarella cheese

Instructions:

1. Place the cheese on the chicken slices and roll them up.

Baked Pumpkin Chips

Ingredients:

- 1 cup of pumpkin, thinly sliced
- 1 tablespoon of olive oil
- Salt and spices to taste

Instructions:

1. Preheat the oven to 400°F (200°C).
2. Toss the pumpkin slices with olive oil and spices.
3. Spread the slices on a baking tray and bake for 20-25 minutes, flipping halfway through.

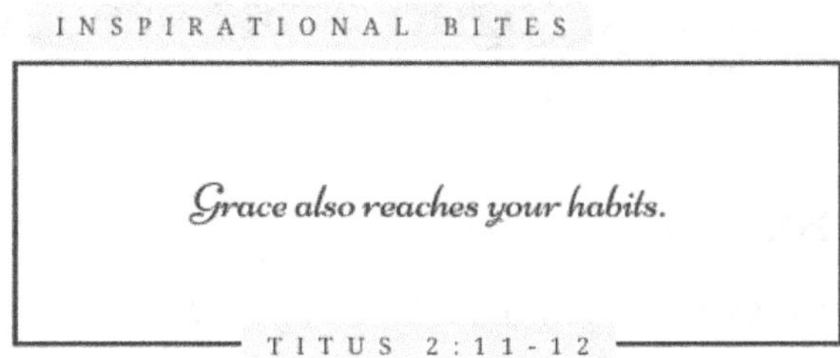

Sugar-Free Gelatin

Ingredients:

• 1 packet of sugar-free gelatin

Instructions:

1. Prepare the gelatin according to the package instructions.
2. Let it cool and refrigerate until set.

Greek Yogurt with Sliced Almonds

Ingredients:

• ½ cup of unsweetened Greek yogurt
• 1 tablespoon of sliced almonds

Instructions:

1. Mix the yogurt with the almonds and serve chilled.

Serrano Ham and Cheese Bites

Ingredients:

- 3 slices of Serrano ham
- 3 pieces of Manchego or Gouda cheese

Instructions:

1. Cut the ham and cheese into small pieces and serve together.

Celery Sticks with Cream Cheese Dip

Ingredients:

• 2 celery stalks, cut into sticks

• 2 tablespoons of cream cheese

Instructions:

1. Serve the celery sticks with the cream cheese as a dip.

Bone Broth Cup

Ingredients:

• 1 cup of natural bone broth

Instructions:

1. Heat the broth in a pot or microwave and serve hot.

Roasted Zucchini Slices with Parmesan Cheese

Ingredients:

- 1 zucchini, sliced
- 2 tablespoons of grated Parmesan cheese

Instructions:

1. Preheat the oven to 400°F (200°C).
2. Place the zucchini slices on a baking tray and sprinkle with Parmesan cheese.
3. Bake for 15 minutes or until golden brown.

Turkey Rolls with Asparagus

Ingredients:

- 2 slices of cooked turkey
- 4 cooked asparagus spears

Instructions:

1. Wrap each asparagus spear with a slice of turkey and serve.

Coconut Flour and Chocolate Mini Muffins

Ingredients (makes 6 small muffins):

• 2 eggs

• 2 tablespoons of coconut flour

• 1 tablespoon of unsweetened cocoa powder

• 1 tablespoon of keto sweetener

Instructions:

1. Preheat the oven to 350°F (180°C).
2. Mix all the ingredients in a bowl.
3. Fill small muffin molds and bake for 12-15 minutes.

Pepperoni Chips

Ingredients:

• 10 slices of pepperoni

Instructions:

1. Preheat the oven to 400°F (200°C).
2. Place the pepperoni slices on a baking tray and bake for 8-10 minutes until crispy.

NOURISHING SMOOTHIES
Drink health. Live with clarity.

Smoothies that Nourish and Sharpen
More than a drink–an intelligent decision

Low-carb smoothies are a practical and delicious way to nourish your body without the sugar overload that affects your energy, focus, and metabolic health. When made with clean ingredients–like leafy greens, healthy fats, and quality proteins–they become powerful allies for stabilizing blood sugar, improving digestion, and extending satiety.

Instead of turning to commercial juices or sugar-filled beverages, these recipes offer real, intentional nutrition. They're perfect as a light breakfast, a revitalizing snack, or even a post-workout boost.

Every sip is an opportunity to honor your body and keep your mind clear.

Energizing Green Smoothie

Ingredients:

- 2 cups of fresh spinach
- 1 ripe avocado
- 2 cups of unsweetened almond milk
- 2 teaspoons of almond butter
- A pinch of cinnamon or a splash of vanilla extract (optional)
- Ice to taste

Instructions:

1. Blend all ingredients until smooth and creamy.
2. Serve chilled.
3. You can garnish with a mint leaf for a refreshing touch.

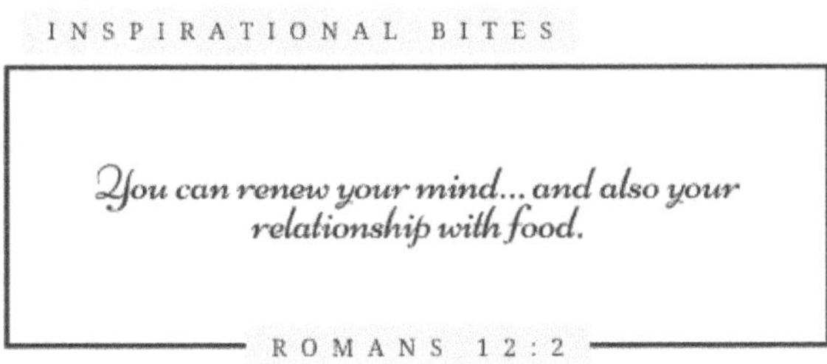

Cacao and Avocado Smoothie

Ingredients:

- 2 cups of unsweetened almond milk
- 2 tablespoons of unsweetened cocoa powder
- 1 ripe avocado
- 1 teaspoon of vanilla extract (optional)
- Natural sweetener to taste (stevia, monk fruit, or dates)
- Ice to taste

Instructions:

1. Blend all ingredients until smooth and silky.
2. Serve with a sprinkle of cinnamon or cocoa powder on top.

Berry and Chia Smoothie

Ingredients:

• 1 cup of frozen berries (strawberries, blueberries, or raspberries)
• 1 tablespoon of chia seeds
• 1 cup of unsweetened coconut or almond milk
• ½ cup of plain unsweetened Greek yogurt
• Natural sweetener to taste
• Ice to taste

Instructions:

1. Blend all ingredients until smooth and creamy.
2. Serve chilled and consume immediately.
3. Shake before drinking if it settles.

Tropical Anti-Inflammatory Smoothie

Ingredients:

• ½ cup of frozen pineapple (optional if you tolerate sweet fruits)

• ½ cup of peeled cucumber

• ½ cup of unsweetened coconut milk

• 1 teaspoon of ground turmeric

• A pinch of black pepper (activates the turmeric)

• Juice of ½ lemon

• Ice to taste

Instructions:

1. Blend everything until fully combined.
2. Serve chilled.
3. This smoothie is perfect for mornings or post-workout recovery.

Coffee & Protein Smoothie

Ingredients:

- 1 cup of cold coffee or espresso
- 1 cup of unsweetened almond milk
- 1 tablespoon of low-carb protein powder
- 1 tablespoon of coconut cream or almond butter
- Ice to taste

Instructions:

1. In a blender, place all ingredients and blend until smooth.
2. Serve as a quick breakfast or an energizing snack.
3. You can sprinkle cinnamon or cocoa on top for a special touch.

Blue Smoothie for Memory Boost

Ingredients:

• ½ cup of frozen blueberries

• 1 cup of cooked and cooled cauliflower (yes, you won't taste it)

• 1 cup of unsweetened coconut or almond milk

• 1 tablespoon of flaxseed or ground flax

• 1 teaspoon of coconut oil or MCT oil

• Natural sweetener to taste

• Ice to taste

Instructions:

1. Blend all ingredients until smooth and creamy.
2. This smoothie is ideal for mornings when you need focus and mental clarity.
3. You can add a touch of cinnamon or nutmeg if desired.

Cucumber and Lemon Detox Smoothie

Ingredients:

• 1 cup of peeled and chopped cucumber

• 1 cup of coconut water or plain water

• Juice of 1 lemon

• 5 fresh mint leaves

• 1 teaspoon of chia seeds (optional)

• Sweetener to taste (if needed)

• Ice to taste

Instructions:

1. Blend all the ingredients until well combined.
2. Serve very cold.
3. This is a refreshing option for after meals or late afternoon–ideal for reducing inflammation and supporting digestion.

TRANSITION, MEAL PREP & PLANNING
Preparing yourself is an act of self-love.

Tips for Transitioning to a Healthier Life

Start where you are, with what you have.

You don't need everything to be perfect to begin. Use what you already have at home and start making small adjustments.

Plan, but stay flexible.

Organization is key, but so is giving yourself grace. If a day doesn't go as planned–don't give up!

Don't punish yourself–educate yourself.

If you slip up, don't see it as failure. Learn from it, identify what triggered it, and return to your path with compassion.

Always have healthy snacks ready.

Hunger-based improvisation is the enemy of focus. Low-carb snacks can save you from poor decisions.

Read labels.

Sugar hides under many names. Knowing what you eat gives you power.

Don't compare your journey.

Everybody is different. What works for others may not work for you. Listen to your body.

Drink water intentionally.

Many times it's not hunger–it's dehydration. Make water a daily ally.

Celebrate progress, not just results.

Did you eat better this week? Sleep better? Have more energy? That matters too!

Do it out of love, not punishment.

This is not about punishing your body–it's about caring for it as the temple it is. Eating well is a way of honoring your life.

You are not alone.

This book is part of a community. Together, we're growing, learning, and focusing. And I, Ive, am celebrating every step with you.

Plan Your Focus

How to Make Prep Meals That Save Time and Decisions

One of the most common reasons we end up eating poorly isn't a lack of knowledge–it's a lack of Instructions. Hunger often strikes without warning, and when there are no ready-to-go options, we tend to choose impulsively, not intentionally.

This is where the power of meal prep comes in. Cooking in advance not only saves time and money–it also protects you from yourself during those moments when you're tired, rushed, or simply starving. Planning your meals allows you to make choices with clarity and care, before emotion or exhaustion speak louder.

A well-nourished body is a focused body. And a solid plan is a tool to avoid chaos and walk with purpose.

Why Do Meal Prep?

• You save money by buying only what you need and avoiding impulse purchases.

• You avoid waste by using what you have strategically.

• You eat better because the decisions were made with a clear mind, not an empty stomach.

• You gain more free time during the week.

• You reduce the stress of deciding what to eat every single day.

Hunger Will Make the Decisions...
If You Don't Make Them First

Behavioral psychology studies show that when the body is in a state of hunger, cortisol levels rise, and the prefrontal cortex (the part of the brain responsible for planning and self-control) is impaired–leading to impulsive rather than rational decisions. This phenomenon is known as *ego depletion* or *decision fatigue.*

A study published in **PNAS** (Proceedings of the National Academy of Sciences, 2011) found that Israeli judges granted more parole early in the day or after breaks, and fewer favorable decisions when hungry or mentally fatigued. Though not directly about food, it illustrates how physical exhaustion and glucose dips lead to more rigid, impulsive, or automatic decisions.

Another study in the **Appetite Journal** (2014) concluded that people experiencing intense hunger tend to choose more calorie-dense foods high in sugar and fat, even when they previously stated a preference for healthier options.

The takeaway? If you don't decide first, hunger will–and it almost never chooses what's best for you.

Weekly Prep Meal Table (for 5 Days)

Category	Prepare on Sunday
Proteins	Cook 2-3 types: chicken, ground beef, hard-boiled eggs
Cooked Vegetables	Sauté or roast spinach, broccoli, bell peppers, zucchini
Raw Vegetables	Chop lettuce, carrots, cucumber, cherry tomatoes
Healthy Fats	Portion out avocado, nuts, oils
Low-Carb Bases	Cauliflower rice, zucchini noodles, mashed cauliflower
Prepared Snacks	Greek yogurt, boiled eggs, sliced cheese
Dressings/Broths	Make a homemade dressing or bone broth

This insight will help you intentionally select the right ingredients for your prep meals and enjoy 5 days of better health and mental clarity.

Smart Shopping Guide

Eat with intention. Shop with purpose.

Planning your grocery shopping is the first step toward eating better, saving money, and staying focused on your goals. Here's a categorized list to support your meal prep, reduce waste, and ensure a variety of nutritious foods throughout the week.

Here's a shopping list to get you started:

Clean and Versatile Proteins

- Chicken breast or thighs
- Ground meat (beef or turkey)
- Eggs
- Canned tuna or salmon in water
- White fish fillets (tilapia, cod)
- Ham, turkey, or roast beef (no added sugar)
- Plain unsweetened Greek yogurt
- Firm tofu or tempeh (optional)

Tip: Cook multiple portions and freeze in individual containers.

Low-Carb Vegetables

• Spinach, kale, Swiss chard

• Broccoli, cauliflower, Brussels sprouts

• Zucchini, cucumber

• Bell peppers (all colors)

• Celery, onion, garlic

• Romaine lettuce, green or purple cabbage

• Asparagus, mushrooms

Tip: Buy fresh veggies for 3-4 days and supplement with frozen vegetables without additives.

Healthy and Functional Fats

• Avocados

• Extra virgin olive oil

• Coconut oil or MCT oil

• Almond or peanut butter (no sugar or added oils)

• Walnuts, almonds, pecans

• Chia, flax, pumpkin, or sunflower seeds

Tip: Store nuts in the refrigerator to preserve their healthy fats.

Low-Sugar Fruits

(In controlled portions)

• Strawberries, blueberries, raspberries

• Lemon and lime

• Unsweetened shredded coconut

• Avocado (yes, it's a fruit 🙂)

Tip: Use them as toppings or in smoothies. Choose unsweetened frozen options.

Pantry Essentials

• Almond flour or coconut flour

• Unsweetened plant-based milk (almond, coconut, cashew)

• Unsweetened cocoa powder

• Low-sodium chicken or vegetable broth

• Low-sodium soy sauce or coconut aminos

• Natural sweeteners: stevia, monk fruit, erythritol

• Apple cider vinegar, mustard, dried herbs and spices

• Natural sofrito (frozen or dehydrated, without added salt)

Tip: Read the labels. Many "healthy" products hide added sugars!

INSPIRATIONAL BITES

What you eat doesn't define you, but it can help you live with more clarity.

MARK 7:15

Useful Frozen Items

- Non-starchy mixed vegetables
- Riced or spiralized cauliflower
- Fish fillets or seafood
- Frozen berries for smoothies
- Frozen fresh herbs (cilantro, basil, parsley)

Hidden Sugars in Foods

Did you know sugar can hide under other names?

Many so-called "healthy" products contain sugar disguised under technical or natural-sounding names. These practices can be misleading and may sabotage your journey toward a low-carb lifestyle.

Knowing these names gives you power when reading labels and helps you make more conscious decisions for your health, focus, and well-being.

Remember: Not everything that *sounds* natural is actually good for your body.

Common Sugar Names on Labels:

Refined Sugars:

• Sugar

• Brown sugar

• Cane sugar

• Inverted sugar

• Turbinado sugar

• Beet sugar

Syrups:

- Corn syrup

- High-fructose corn syrup (HFCS)

- Maple syrup

- Rice syrup

- Malt syrup

- Flavored syrups: caramel, chocolate, strawberry

Fructose and Derivatives:

- Fructose

- Fruit juice concentrate

- Evaporated cane juice

- Agave nectar

- Coconut nectar

Other Technical Names:

- Dextrose

- Maltose

- Glucose

- Sucrose

- Lactose (natural sugar in milk)

- Maltodextrin (*very common in "fitness" snacks*)

- Galactose

Important Tip for You:

If you spot more than one type of sugar on the ingredient list–
even in small amounts–**watch out!** The product may have a
high glycemic index, even if it claims to have "no added sugar."

Easy Substitution List

Mindful eating isn't about perfection – it's about intention.

On the journey to healthier eating, we often stop when we're missing an ingredient, don't know how to replace it, or feel like if we don't follow the recipe exactly, it "doesn't count."
But it doesn't have to be that way.

Flexibility is key to consistency.

This list was created to help you keep moving forward–even when your pantry isn't perfect. Because it's not about having everything, it's about doing the best you can with what you have. Each suggested swap is designed to maintain the nutritional balance of your meals without sacrificing flavor or purpose.

- When you have options, you don't get stuck.
- When you understand the *why* behind your choices, you don't lose motivation.
- When you eat with focus, you don't eat on impulse.

So, keep this guide close. Use it anytime you feel short on resources or ideas.

Remember: Eating with intention isn't rigidity–it's freedom with direction.

Practical Tips:

• Don't get frustrated. Flexibility is part of sustainable success.
• Adjust liquids. If your substitute is drier or thicker, add more liquid as needed.
• Trust your taste buds. Substitutions are also a great way to discover new flavors.

If You Don't Have... | Use Instead...

Almond flour	Coconut flour (use only 1/3 the amount and add 1 extra egg)
Avocado	Greek yogurt or coconut cream (for smoothies or creaminess)
Egg	1 tablespoon ground flaxseed + 3 tablespoons water (let sit 5 min)
Almond/peanut butter	Tahini, sunflower seed butter, or cashew butter
Cauliflower	Grated zucchini, finely chopped broccoli, or cabbage
Spinach	Kale (without stems), Swiss chard, or mixed lettuce greens
Ground meat	Ground chicken, ground turkey, or cooked lentils (vegetarian option)
Low-carb bread	Lettuce leaves, cabbage, or egg wraps
Sugar or honey	Stevia, monk fruit, or erythritol
Mayonnaise	Plain Greek yogurt or mashed avocado
Cream cheese	Whipped cottage cheese or ricotta

Pasta or rice	Zoodles (spiralized zucchini), cauliflower rice, or sautéed cabbage strips
Fresh sofrito	Dried sofrito or quick mix of chopped onion, garlic, peppers, and cilantro
Potatoes	Rutabaga, chayote, or jicama
Regular milk	Almond, coconut, or walnut milk
Coconut flour	Ground flaxseed or a seed blend
Unsweetened almond milk	Light coconut milk, cashew milk, or water + nut butter
Plain Greek yogurt	Cottage cheese, plain kefir, or unsweetened sour cream

||

Frequently Asked Questions

1. What if I want rice or bread?

You don't have to give them up forever, but you can make smarter swaps like cauliflower rice or low-carb bread. If you choose to have a small portion of brown rice or sourdough bread, pair it with plenty of vegetables and protein to avoid blood sugar spikes.

2. Can I eat fruit?

Yes, in moderation. Prioritize low-sugar fruits like strawberries, blueberries, raspberries, lemon, and unsweetened coconut. Avoid juices and dried fruits, which pack a lot of sugar into a small portion.

3. What if I mess up one day?

You didn't fail–you simply made a choice. This is not a journey of perfection but of awareness. Come back to your focus without guilt and keep going. Every meal is a new opportunity.

4. Can I do this if my family eats differently?

Absolutely! You can prepare a common base (proteins and vegetables) and add carbs separately for those who want them. Over time, your family will notice the benefits in you– and they may want to try it too.

5. Do I have to obsess over counting carbs?

No. If you eat real, unprocessed foods focused on vegetables, healthy fats, and clean proteins, you'll naturally reduce your carb intake. What matters most is quality–not obsession.

6. How long does it take to see results?

Many people feel more energy, better digestion, and fewer cravings in the first week. Others take longer. Every body is unique. Be patient with yourself and observe the process with love.

7. What can I do if I crave sweets?

Try a smoothie, drink lemon water, go for a walk, pray, or take deep breaths. Many cravings are more emotional than physical. Remember your "why" and reconnect with yourself.

8. What can I take with me when I go out?

A handful of nuts, boiled eggs, homemade low-carb bars, or even a smoothie in a thermos. Preparing ahead is a way of caring for yourself. Don't improvise when you're hungry.

9. Can I do this during perimenopause or menopause?

Yes–and it's highly recommended! Lowering carbs helps stabilize hormones, reduce inflammation, and prevent the energy crashes that are common during this stage.

10. Is this a diet?

No. It's a mindset shift. It's a way of eating with intention, making peace with your body, and making choices that move you closer to the full health you deserve.

Conclusion

It's not just about what you eat–it's about how you choose to live.

You've reached the end of this 30-day journey, but in truth, you're beginning something much deeper: a life of greater awareness, energy, and focus.

This book is not a diet. It's a guide to awaken your intention. To remind you that your body is not a failed project–but a temple full of potential.

Every decision you make–every balanced breakfast, every light dinner, every smoothie full of life–is a way to reconnect with your purpose, your health, and your mental and spiritual well-being.

Cutting sugar is not just about what you're giving up–it's about everything you gain:
Clarity, peace, vitality, self-control, and a sharper mind to live out the calling God placed in you.

"Self-control is more than willpower–it is a fruit of the Spirit." (Galatians 5:22-23)

If you've made it this far, I want you to remember this:

You can.

Your mind can be renewed.

Your body can heal.

Your focus can grow stronger.

And you are not alone. I'm right here with you–celebrating every step.

Keep walking this path with love–not perfection, but direction.

With love,

Chef Ive Adorno

A Boricua in Ohio

Acknowledgments

To my husband Fran, thank you...

For reading this book more times than anyone could imagine.

For caring about every single word with me, making sure everything was clear, useful, and doable.

For your patience when I lost mine.

For your support when I felt like I couldn't go on.

For tasting every recipe–even the ones that didn't turn out as we hoped.

And for reminding me every day that this project had value, because it was born from love.

This book is yours too.

To Gladys, my mom, thank you for being that gentle but firm voice that always pushed me forward.

For encouraging me when moving forward felt impossible, and for reminding me, with faith, that what is born with purpose always comes to fruition in due time.

To you, who chose to change your eating habits to be with us longer.

This book is our baby–nearly a year in the making.

A year of doubts, ideas, tweaks, and recipes.

But also a year sustained by love, family, faith–and above all, by God, who called me to write.

Thank you for always being there.

About the Author

Ivelisse Adorno, known as **Chef Ive Adorno**, is a proud *Boricua in Ohio*–a daughter of God, wife, author, certified coach, neurotheologian, speaker, and Christian entrepreneur passionate about holistic transformation.

In 2020, after contracting COVID-19, she faced a severe health crisis that nearly cost her life. What followed was an intense battle with anxiety, brain fog, and physical and spiritual exhaustion.

That season marked the beginning of a deep rebuilding process–of her health, her faith, her mind... and her purpose. With God's help and a firm decision to heal, she began studying a master's degree in neurotheology, discovering how faith, nutrition, and intentional thinking can activate the healing and focus that both body and soul need.

This book is not just a cookbook; it's part of her testimony. A guide for those who long to eat with intention, heal from within, and rediscover the focus lost in the haze of exhaustion and sugar.

She has published several books, including the successful **"Mis Recetas Favoritas de Quinoa," "Nutre tu Cuerpo y tu Cerebro,"** and the devotional **"Mujeres de Negocios, Mujeres de Fe."**

She also leads **Kitvi Editorial, LLC**, her Christian publishing house, coaches' entrepreneurial women, and runs **Ruta 333 Travel**, a travel agency that proves a fulfilling life *is* possible.

She lives in Ohio with her husband Fran–her love, kitchen, and travel companion.

Did You Enjoy This Book? There's More for You!

Thank you for letting me accompany you on this journey toward intentional eating.

If this book inspired you, I'm sure you'll also enjoy other titles I've written–with the same heart and holistic focus on mind, body, and spirit:

• <u>Quinoa con Sazón Boricua</u>

Easy, flavorful, and healthy recipes that celebrate our roots with a modern twist.

• <u>Nourish Your Brain and Body</u>

Simple recipes to help you reconnect with your body, establish new habits, and move forward with self-love and clarity.

• **Businesswomen of Faith**

A powerful devotional for entrepreneurial women who want to walk with God in every decision.

If any of these titles speak to you, you can find them on Amazon under my name or at:

🌐 <u>www.iveadorno.com</u>

Thank You for Reading

Less Sugar, More Focus

Thank you for making it this far!

If you've completed this 30-day journey, we celebrate with you.

This book was written with love, intention, and purpose... and now, it carries your story too.

Did this book help you?

Your experience can inspire others.

If it was a blessing to you, please:

Leave us an honest review on Amazon.

Your voice helps others discover this resource.

Special Thanks

To you, dear reader, for trusting this process.

And to everyone walking toward a healthier, clearer, and more purposeful life:

Thank you for inspiring us!